Before They Left Us

Rosemary Ann Davis

Our bodies spun
On swivels of bone & faith,
Through a lyric slipknot
Of Joy, & we knew we were
Beautiful & dangerous.

—Yusef Komunyakaa

ISBN: 978-1-7322845-0-0 (paperback)
    978-1-7322845-2-4 (hardcover)
    978-1-7322845-1-7 (e-book)

Visit
www.rosemaryanndavis.com
for more information about the author

Published by
Old Road Publishing
Minneapolis, Minnesota

San Francisco itself is art, above all literary art.
Every block is a short story, every hill a novel.
Every home a poem, every dweller within
immortal. That is the whole truth.

—William Saroyan

In memory of John, Paul, Howard,
Neal, Casey, Malcolm, James, Rosemary,

and so many others.

Acknowledgments

My deepest thanks to Barrie Jean Borich and Lawrence Sutin for their guidance.

Writer, editor John D'Agata and NAMES Project AIDS Quilt Founder Cleve Jones for their expertise and support.

Gordon Thomas for manuscript evaluation and developmental editing.

Dara Syrkin for structural advice and proofing.

Patti Frazee for transcription and consulting.

My memoir, poetry, and travel writing groups for their endless encouragement.

Personal thanks to Diane Delesha, Laurie Pouchak, Elinor Auge, Ellen Shriner, Catherine Watson, Michael Kiesow Moore, and the late Marty Wright for their friendship. Loren Hooyman for mentoring. Kim and Elizabeth for their feedback and love.

Eileen Beha and Grey Guindon for convincing me to publish.

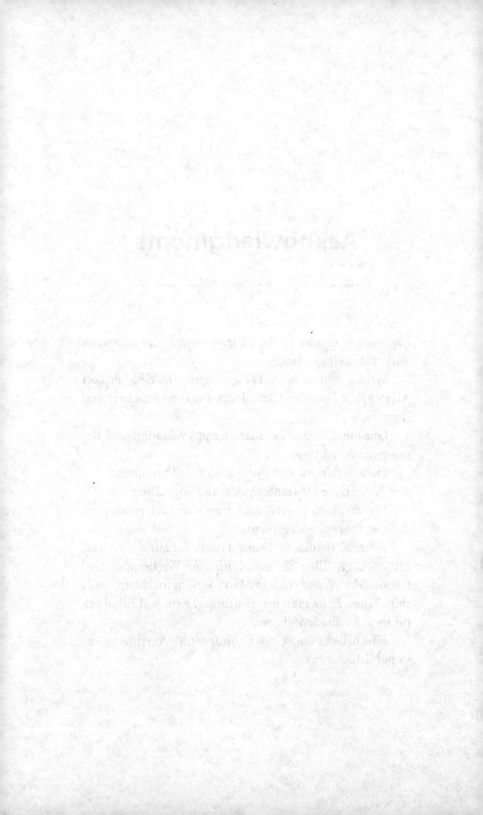

Prologue

Cemetery

Click, click. Breathe. I hold my camera lens steady between the spokes of an iron gate fronting a funeral chamber. From my viewfinder, I see a small masonry room. A stone shelf holds a graceful vase shaped like a swan. Inside the swan, an array of flowers emerge wilted. Roses. Carnations. Baby's breath. I've never liked daisies or other common flowers, but for some reason the carnations don't bother me here. Their stems bend and twist into a silent design, awaiting the hand of a painter. What I'm capable of at this moment is laying the scene onto film. The decayed flora and the fine delicacy of a spiderweb provide the only softness in a room of stone, the only still life offerings. Yet there is my breath, which now seeps into this space. I blink, and for a second, everything goes black.

Death fascinates me. Always has, although back then I hadn't yet lost many people in my life. At my grandfather's funeral, the assembled clan laughed heartily and drank too much. This so mystified me as an adolescent. Not the drinking too much—that was a given. It was their laughter that startled me. I asked my father, "How can these people be laughing? This is so sad." His knowing response came as we took shelter in the Milwaukee funeral parlor doorway, he laying his arm across my scant shoulder. "Yes, they do care. But if they didn't laugh, they'd all be crying."

His statement offered a deep philosophical insight into my family, one I could not fully grasp as I watched them interact. As an adolescent, the interactions with inebriated aunts and uncles at social functions disturbed me so much that I made an internal promise to steer clear of my extended family whenever possible.

The window above the swan washes the space with daylight, save the old-fashioned portrait of Jesus in a wooden frame hiding in shadow near the ceiling. He gazes down, his sacred heart exposed. I didn't notice that on either side of the symmetrical design of this room were the beginnings of the name "Catherine" etched into the wall on the right, and a part of a birth date—the twenty-fifth day in December, Christmas Day in the 1870s. On the left, a last name is not completely legible except for the letters OMPAGNO. Perhaps Catherine's husband, who died on March 28, 1949, rests here? The dates, outlining several lives, crawl magnificently across the surfaces. When I examined the photograph later, I noticed the name and periods of time, but while in that spare, impossibly still space, my eyes and curiosity were fixated on what lay directly in front of me—the religious icon, the flowers placed in memorial by a visitor long ago, and the sunlight.

This private mausoleum is the first photograph I developed and printed on my own in a photo class I took when first arriving in the Bay Area. I knew that although I was part of a group of fellow photographers, my quest to record images was ultimately a solitary endeavor. Like my aunts and uncles, the other students resided in the outer perimeters of my consciousness. I shot thirty-six images that afternoon in the hilltop California cemetery in 1975. Looking at the proof sheet, I see the images in miniature—fractured tablet headstones, rosette window, and a marker for a Baby Elizabeth, which I had stroked gently with my hand, perhaps knowing even then that I would remain childless. Various other graves peer out from the high weeds, contained by wooden or metal fencing, most in the state of disrepair either through relentlessness of wind, the disregard of vandals, or the sheer weight of time.

Catherine's resting place captured all of the elements that intrigued me: beauty, tragedy, history, and simplicity. Here was an intimate place where a presence remained. The distance between Catherine and me measures more than one hundred years, two pieces of glass (my lens and the window to her tomb), and my curiosity. Who was she? And who is that young woman looking back at her?

The only time I saw my father cry was after his father died. He sat at the kitchen table, his head in his hands, and sobbed. I probably wasn't supposed to see this, but I'm glad I did. Perhaps it prepared me in some small way for understanding death and the grief that accompanies it. I saw my father as a vulnerable, very human adult, without his usual masks of humor or stoicism. He sat alone at the kitchen table that night, shirtless, his hands covering his face. I just stood there in the doorway and watched him cry.

In time, I was able to view my aunts and uncles with compassion, as I, too, began to understand my own faults and shortcomings.

I could have stayed on that Oakland hill indefinitely, walking near the knotted trees and between the bent headstones, past some overgrown burial sites and tilted crosses, up close to the old photographs fastened to monuments, near stone statues of favorite saints. I wanted to document this place, remember it, perhaps revisit it from time to time.

Prophetically so, I have done exactly that over the course of my life. Although a wild garden of daffodils sprang up in vivid yellows, I photographed in black and white. Even in the bright sun, the tones are rich, showing a contrast between the lighter and darker shades. Exquisite architectural details reveal themselves in between the film's sprockets, the landscape pushes itself forward, and the spirits of many people, all unknown to me, rise.

Discover

_____

Here We Are

Actually, I'm not in this one. I must have taken the photograph. Or was I not there at all? Anyway, here we are—the group. We're in the kitchen at 364 Sanchez. I can't tell who is living in the apartment now. Is it Kim and Jon? Oh, it must be, because when Neal and John were together, it was in the mid-1970s. Okay. It is Kim and Jon's kitchen. Everyone is standing at the counter. There is some kind of salad on a plate, perhaps a makeshift tuna, my favorite. Next to it is the breadboard with a sliced baguette. An empty glass. I wonder if we ate after the pictures were taken.

In the first picture, everyone is standing or sitting up straight, looking rather serious and posed in front of the refrigerator. Jon is very young here; I didn't know him well then. He's got brown hair in the photo. Now, he's bald. His dark shirt with the striped collar is open; he is looking straight into the camera with his right hand extended toward the curtains with the wild pink and green flowers. Casey, my old roommate, is next. Her arms are crossed on the counter, a slight smile on her youthful face.

Neal towers over everyone, including Casey, whom he is slightly behind. She's relaxed, always ready with a joke. His white shirt is open, his arm resting on the back of Paul's chair. Kim, in her short-cropped hair and Southern charm held in check, is barely visible behind Paul, who is sitting in the chair, his red hair, mustache (oh, I miss him), his left arm straight down and hand braced on the seat. John's arm touches Paul's shoulder. Those two were inseparable friends. I miss John too. He was my best friend. Here, he is in a dark jean jacket, the other hand in his pants pocket, plaid shirt, trimmed mustache, short hair, kind eyes—they are all focused on me and the camera. That is, *if* I was there.

In the second photo, pandemonium! The pose completely disrupted because they thought the picture taking was done. Casey bursts into laughter. Paul is caught half-kneeling and jumping out of his chair, his muscular arms pushing himself upward, finally less serious. John, standing apart, shimmers in soft focus. Kim, one arm bent at her waist, the other covering her mouth, while Neal, in the back, heartily claps.

Whim

Thirty-two years ago, I moved to San Francisco and landed (thanks to the referral from an old boyfriend) in a Victorian house situated on the panhandle of Golden Gate Park. It was home to a couple of carpet-cleaning musicians, and me with enough naiveté to qualify as the sibling of a tie-dyed flower child. At twenty-three, this seemed better than the place I'd been before, not just because of the weather, but because it offered so much more culture. San Francisco presented me with a larger array of choices for jobs, housing, and entertainment. And most important, it provided me the freedom to really be myself and to explore my creative side.

In my hometown of Milwaukee, a place where the word "work" was a mantra, "art" tempted me but remained untouchable. In the Bay Area, the arts flourished—plays, concerts, opera, dance— and this made my eyes pop, drawing me inside various doors and making me feel like a native. I stood on a high hill in the Castro area and looked down on the streets below, liking the way the Victorians lined up: all high and mighty, and yet grounded. As if waiting for me to walk by.

I could readily eavesdrop on conversations in Mandarin and Spanish, taste fresh artichokes and cilantro, and smell scattered camellias, which I pressed between pages of my books. I moved to San Francisco because it seemed no greater a decision than most I'd made in my short adult life, and even then I had learned to trust myself, so when the notion presented itself after a short trip there, I rather logically thought about it over coffee on the airplane home. Well, why not move to San Francisco? It seemed like a good idea at the time (and I pondered it as I did many options at that age, with a weighing of the pros and cons). The decision had arrived by the time I disembarked the plane. I moved to San Francisco on a very strong whim. Thank God.

What It Was Really Like

The year was 1975, long before I knew how hip it was to live in San Francisco, and longer still before Bin Laden warned of blowing up its bridges. My gang converged—a bustling, robust clan of straight and gay alike who bonded and lived large during the last years before AIDS. To be sure, the times were the pinnacle of an excessive, drug-induced, musically inspired funfest. But these were real people, I among them, and we used the city as a playground. We went to free concerts at Stern Grove, wandered along Stinson Beach on warm afternoons, hiked the woods of Mount Tamalpais on holidays, and ate huge beef and bean burritos from Valencia Street whenever we had the chance. We were in our twenties and had no authority figures to boss us around. San Francisco was made for the young; still is. When I was young, we came from all other parts of the country—East, South, and Midwest—just to be here.

San Francisco was everything I'd ever heard about it—steep hills, expansive bridges, the most crooked street in the world, palm trees. Cable cars turned around daily, down by the Woolworth store, where friends had their pictures taken. It was the only photo booth in the city, which shot in black-and-white film. Cherry blossoms rested on wooden arbors deep in the Japanese Tea Garden in Golden Gate Park. Diebenkorn's paintings hung at the Museum of Modern Art and ninety-year-old Imogen Cunningham's photographs, along with her stamina, caught my eye. Rows of painted ladies, Victorian houses, filled with ferns. Sourdough bread, fresh crab, and a nice bottle of California table wine—one for each visitor. For residents, even the newest ones like me, California's gifts were so much deeper.

Home

Of the many places I called home in San Francisco during the 1970s, all were close to the Castro neighborhood. Whether it was a duplex on Thirtieth and Church, filled with a crowd of Philly roommates, an apartment on Guerrero with a woman who shared my first name, the flat above the Chinese grocery on Sanchez, where I lived with a bookie, or the one off Dolores Park (formerly inhabited by a musician in the NBC band), all roads led to Castro.

At one point, I had seven very close gay male friends, but not all of them knew each other. My straight femaleness turned me into almost every man's kid sister, amusing buddy, or someone to ignore. I also knew a number of women and straight couples, although far fewer. Living among hundreds of homosexuals for years led me to not only accept the culture, but to look at straight couples as oddities.

On the intersection of Eighteenth and Castro stood the Bank of America, followed by the Spaghetti Factory, and up a few steps, a comfortable bookstore and a breakfast place with hidden garden seating inside. The food wasn't that great, but the atmosphere proved just fine for Sunday brunch. Sometimes I stopped at the tiny oyster bar, which looked more like a diner. Across the street was the Elephant Walk Bar (our own version of New York's Stonewall), where the cops stormed in one night and beat the living crap out of all the gay male patrons.

Yes, I did get quite an education. I learned about the encounters that took place in that bookstore at the end of my block, what went on in the bathhouses, and where the teenage hustlers stood as soon as the sun went down. It both fascinated and disturbed me. The randomness of men's loving was not all that different from my own. I enjoyed sex my first night in the Bay Area and never looked back. Since venereal diseases were considered a minor inconvenience in those days, sexual pleasures were unlimited. No regrets. No apologies. Gay or straight.

Church Street

Casey picked me. Of all the people coming up those worn brown steps to be interviewed, I was the one she said yes to. I became the new roommate and the Church Street flat became my first home in San Francisco.

Casey was intense. Like me, she was young and she was funny. God, was she funny. Wickedly. A Catholic schoolgirl from New Jersey, she talked fast and with a confidence that belied her age. She was about twenty-five, long brown hair, skinny body. Casey was one wild young woman.

Among the many jobs she had—waitress in a soup kitchen, manager of a hot tub spa, and others—she also (unbeknownst to her roommates) worked as a bookie out of our Victorian flat. We got our first inkling of her extra "job" while in a restaurant, where we were seated next to a table of cops. Casey started to break out in a sweat and later that night she told us. I remember worrying that our house could be raided at any time and we would all be rounded up. Luckily, that didn't happen.

Despite her illegal occupation, I looked up to and admired her. She may have appeared tough and fearless, but she also had a nurturing side—bringing soup for dinner when one of us was sick, taking in a Chinese woman and her baby who had nowhere to go.

Casey introduced me to her friends, who then became my friends, and so it went.

Home for us was a second-floor flat out on Twenty-Ninth and Church, which is the end of the line for the J Church. The streetcar turned and repeated its path just beyond our street. Prominent in our neighborhood were St. Luke's Catholic church and grade school. The school had a large blacktop playground, where Casey and I went to shoot hoops. Streets nearby held a Chinese corner store, a bakery, and a fresh fruit and vegetable market.

Our flat was rather nondescript, except for its stunning view. Out the front window I could see the decoratively carved woodwork fronting the house next door. The blond cornices looked stunning to the young woman I was becoming, who had dreamt of being a carpenter but never made it past the first class. The view out the back revealed a classic framed barn situated behind a neighbor's Victorian.

While I always believed that the views were the best part and the inside of our place too plain, it did provide ample room for the group of us who resided there. I came to live in this flat after responding to a roommate-wanted ad through the Women's Switchboard, where I worked as a crisis call volunteer when I first moved to San Francisco.

After the inaugural Irish coffee at the Buena Vista Café, I was off listening and dancing to Irish bands, volunteering, and searching for a job.

Downtown

Heading downtown to the Financial District for the first time, I stare out the streetcar window. When the landscape changes and the buildings grow much taller, I jump off. This is well before I should have. Before the cable car turns around at Powell and Market Streets, next to the Woolworth's. Before the big department stores. Before Union Square, where the famous mimes perform. And before the elegant Garden Court of the Palace Hotel, where I will one day enjoy brunch with women friends. Before the Financial District, where my job will be, and Chinatown that follows. No, I have gotten off too soon. I do not know that yet, however.

I step onto the wide street and look around. Sleazy movie theaters and storefronts smack up against each other with metal gratings their owners roll up and down at will. Tables outside hold cheaply made electronics, T-shirts, and various tchotchkes. Barkers hawking anything they can. I am out of my element. Dirty sidewalks, loud boom boxes—not what I expected.

I don't know anyone well here, but that doesn't matter. It seems that many are from somewhere else, or have just arrived, like myself. The hippies, yuppies, and homeless seem to coexist in harmony. San Francisco is far more diverse than Milwaukee, with people from every country in the world. At this point, I'm just a student of the city, studying it all. This education proves to be both exhilarating and frightening. San Francisco is like any other place I don't know—foreign territory. It will take days, weeks, and months to get a grasp of the lay of the land and to make friends. I leave my suitcase out, ready for a quick exit if it becomes necessary.

Even in my hometown in the Midwest, I felt alone. People have often mistaken my solitary existence for something grim, but that's not the case. My aloneness is my solace. I want to make connections with others but also want to protect my inner space, the place where I inhabit my thoughts and ruminate about what comes next in my ever-evolving life.

In these early days of adjusting to my new life in San Francisco, I'm content to observe. To look out windows of a streetcar, to cross a boundary between neighborhoods, to find the courage to call another stranger on the list of names I compiled from friends in other places. My voice cracks a bit as I throw out a line to the other side: "Karen suggested I call you. I just moved to the Bay Area, and I'm wondering if you have time for a coffee? By the way, do you know a good place to go dancing?"

Back on Market Street, I see a familiar sign.

I approach McDonald's like an old friend. I order breakfast. Sitting at a table with my food, I look up to see a nearby table crowded with women. On closer inspection of their wiry bodies, scant clothing, and unruly hair, I realize they are hookers. My discomfort shows and as I hurriedly eat my Egg McMuffin, I notice the girls vying to get a look at me. They laugh. I feel myself shaking. I must look so green. Blue jeans and T-shirt, long brown hair with premature white stripes. No makeup. I don't know anyone here and have no idea where I am going. I hear their laughter as I flee to the street.

Bright Clouds

Bright clouds ferret away the last glimpses of the sun. Gay men jam the sidewalks, while a song of Donna Summer's can be heard coming from a car radio. When a tourist bus bounces past, local residents, including me, stop and wave. The pizza is hot across the street from the Castro Theatre, where a double bill of Marlene Dietrich is playing. All this among the cherry blossoms of the Japanese Tea Garden, the bold tower of the Transamerica Pyramid, and the persistent hum of cable cars making their final turnaround at Powell and Market.

Cable Cars

Cable cars roamed the hills—no, rather, they jumped and clanged and attacked the hills around Chinatown and into the neighborhoods near the downtown shopping areas almost around the clock. They spun around in circles near Powell and Market, where tourists waited giddily in long lines to board them.

The drivers, a boisterous group of independents, acted the part with finesse. With planted berets, they roused the crowd by dramatically ringing the bell. I sat on these cars as well. Once it was new to me, when I cautiously reached my seat on the outside of the car and discovered it faced the street directly. I sat with wide eyes and waited for a new kind of ride.

The car jerked forward and with that I swallowed. The uneven pull of it yanking us along California Street on the edge of the Fillmore District could be terrifying or gleeful. The bell rang out, and people got off and on at will. Some streets were the traditional hills of the area, while others were smooth and flat; but it was the curves that were the most thrilling, especially when matched by the speed of the rickety cars.

Tourists took the cable cars so they could tell their pals that they had done it. The cars brought them en masse and deposited them at Fisherman's Wharf, a major tourist attraction. This area contained seafood restaurants, Cost Plus, various gift shops, and fishing operations, such as places where you could watch the crab crackers work. The young men would toss the fish back and forth— it was live theater.

Near the wharf rested Ghirardelli Square, where folks could buy the famous chocolate, gather unique paper kites, and dip into an art gallery if they liked.

The best time for residents to ride the streetcars to arrive at the wharf would be on a weeknight. This way they could avoid the tourists. And we would never go there on a weekend; it would just be too crowded. Now that I lived here, my tourist days were over.

Yet the adventures continued, taking me on a twisty, curvy ride, unimaginable at the time.

Meeting

As my circle of friends continued to expand, I was invited to parties and dinners, especially through Casey and her social circles. One night, I went to a barbecue (against my better judgment, for I was sick with the flu), where I met an assortment of Casey's friends, including two gay men named John and Paul. Both were from the East Coast and had arrived in California a few years before I had. They worked at Stone Soup on the line together and also shared a flat. John, in his jeans and fedora, was dating a man named Neal, also from New York. Paul was on his own. These two were so funny that, even though I was quite sick, they had me rolling with laughter. Paul would turn toward us and in an exaggerated accent say, "I love the Ayatollah." In the following days, I plotted how I would see them again. Luckily, there would be a party at their place the next weekend. They were the first gay men that I ever really knew. It wasn't long before they pulled me into their circle, keeping me there for years.

Redheaded Paul was quite handsome and zen, which appealed to me. I wondered if he was bisexual. He was rather shy but had the most biting sense of humor. "I can't believe that you were actually able to make it out here on your own," Paul told me once. I, too, was bashful in the beginning but quickly gained confidence after I started college and began making friends.

John, with his shaggy brown hair and small frame, was the perfect man to play Charlie Chaplin at Halloween. He was kind and friendly, loved to cook, and was giving haircuts to all of his friends. Gardens, pets—he was a nurturing kind of guy. In time, he nurtured me.

They both did.

Also in that group were Kim and Mark, a couple of friends who had come from the South and dazzled us with their graceful charm and dramatic overtures. Watching them was like witnessing performance art. Kim and Mark went on to star in one of my student films, as did John and Paul. We drew each other closer into the things that were important to us.

We all became friends over time and I joined their Stone Soup circle, staying with them long after I moved out of that flat and after each of them had made their way beyond soups and sandwiches.

Working, going to school, and being part of an expansive group of friends were more important to me than what most young women my age were doing—getting married. I saw myself as out in the world and not stuck in a house like my mother. There were no "parents" in this town, I soon discovered, so I pushed myself creatively with photography and filmmaking and, like many around me, tentatively explored the nuances of my sexuality and expanded my friendships into the gay community.

Moccasins

"John, is this the way this stitch is supposed to look?"

"Here, let me take a look at that. Yeah, that's right. You've got it."

I sighed. These moccasins were taking a lot longer to make than I thought they would. First, we measured the feet of the folks who would be wearing them. In my case, they were for my dad. We then shopped for the materials, bought good-sized leather scraps, something for the soles, special needles to sew with, glue, and some lacing.

Each week for several months we took a nighttime drive to Half Moon Bay and received lessons from a woman there. This rounded woman would come to the door to usher us in, like an auntie on craft night. We'd haul in our supplies and receive the next instructions before driving home in the dark. I'd cut my strips of the material according to the pattern. So would John. The moccasins were one of many projects that we took on together. Next we built wooden racks for our pots and pans. Making things—we liked to keep busy. We liked working with our hands. These undertakings were tactile, challenging, and gave us a sense of accomplishment.

Peanuts & Beer

Peanuts. Two beers each and peanuts. Every Tuesday night at my place. The doorbell would ring three times in rapid succession (our code) at exactly 7:30 p.m. I'd let him in. Paul stopped by after his job making solicitation phone calls for a political newsletter, or so he said. Days found him in school. His major was psychology, and often on Tuesday nights we'd discuss various types of therapy and mental illness. At that time, I was seeing a psychologist named Sherry. Her office was off the N Judah streetcar line, near the creamery. Paul heard about all of our weekly sessions. You could say that he was my *other* therapist. Not a good cop versus bad cop scenario—they were both good. His listening skills were excellent and Paul would make a fine psychologist himself. His goal was to work with gay youth. His future clients would love him—hysterically funny, sensitive, and honest.

Paul and I talked about self-help books, famous psychologists, and our own problems. I listened to how he had lost his virginity and stories of different men he had met at the bars. Then it was my turn to tell him about the men I had met at the bars. Neither of us could ever settle down to just one partner. We took all of our discussions very seriously, even though we used our humor and cynicism sometimes to approach sensitive areas. We were confiding in each other the most intimate details of our twenty-five years of life and also sharing our interest in analysis—the process and the practice.

I thought of Paul as a soul mate. We danced together in the supermarket, had make-believe fights in public, and once when I had gone out to a party, he scaled the front of my apartment building to get through my open window so he could let a crowd inside to see the Rolling Stones on *Saturday Night Live*. When I returned home to this scene, I just laughed.

Paul could be shy at times; he was an introvert at heart. Sarcastic. Brutally honest. I couldn't tell which trait was worse (or best). When he thought deeply, he would reach up with his finger and rub his mustache. I don't think he even knew he did it. For that matter, I used to blink a lot when I was nervous, so what's the difference? They were just the quirks of our young selves.

———————

More peanuts. Another beer?

These Tuesday night sessions went on for three years. And our friendship grew.

My Place

An ornate metal grating shelters the entrance, its focus straight ahead, fighting the urge to lean into an angle mimicking the street. I turn the key. The brass mailboxes beckon as they have for decades, then the weighted front door. The lobby—reminiscent of a Diane Arbus photo—winds long and dark. Decked with artificial foliage, it leads to the stairs. At the top, I find the door—my new door—and enter. The landlord gives permission to move in early, if I clean the place myself. Wood floors, worn but functional, carry me from hall to cavernous living room to bay window. Dolores Park unfolds before me. Mission High School anchors the bottom of the hill, the green sliding straight up for two blocks, my apartment situated a third of the way, streetcars visible from the window, along with palms, men walking hand in hand, all graced by the song of mourning doves.

Stepping away from the living room bay window, I pass through the double french doors to the bedroom—very dark when I first take possession of the apartment. I grab hold of some old curtains and bring them down. Beyond that is a flimsy plastic shower curtain, beneath which is a thick layer of yellowed newspaper taped to the huge window to keep the world out. It comes down as well. Behind the glass, an air well, interesting enough to be photographed at a later date, but now, aside from being a still life, it sends in rays of filtered light that make the room habitable. From my new bed, only the brightened white dome of one of Mission High School's towers fills my view. Gazing upon it, I feel like I am in Greece.

In the kitchen, a booth with built-in benches takes the corner, the cupboards keep their original wooden backboard, and I gaze with awe at the stove. The Occidental, which has a large griddle to the left and wood-burning cavity to the right, is a gem. Despite being a non-cook, I sense my eyes widen, my mouth gape. The previous occupant, a musician in the NBC band, lived here only three months a year, the time when he was not on tour. When I first saw the space, it was stacked with his books and papers, not to mention those awful layered window coverings. Now only the last meal, still sitting in the oven (something burnt and definitely petrified), and a few posters of his Chinese heritage remain.

I paint the living room with a refrigerator drawer full of burgundy paint. The voracious walls soak up the pigment but still loom large. The french doors are done twice, first in white—too stark—then in tan—easier on the eye. The floors I steel wool, buff, and seal, while the bedroom transforms as white on white to brighten the darkness preferred by its previous occupant. Later, when I make love in that room with a man named Philip, he glances around with his painter's eye and admires the two tones of white, as if I, too, am an artist.

I find vintage forest-green wallpaper in a neighborhood paint store and slide it up with my hands above the kitchen booth. Finally, dozens of knobs, bolts, racks, and various parts I know nothing about come off the stove. I meticulously clean and return them to their rightful places. The apartment becomes filled with ferns, stuffed old furniture, deep rugs, and a print of black patrons from Milwaukee dancing in a North Side nightclub.

This place, the only space in my San Francisco journey that is all mine (*only* mine), gives me a big, broad playground to work in, to create from, and to dwell in. I can break the simple rules of a conventional upbringing by painting the largest room red, by sleeping in the white bedroom with various partners, by dabbling with intoxicants in the kitchen, and knowing the footprint of this home so well that I can find the bathroom in the dark. I can fill it with art of my liking, huge spider plants and ferns, furniture from

Noe Valley, where a junk dealer has similar taste, and with friends, ones I'll know for the long haul. Or so I thought.

I furnish it with meticulous care to detail, including the furniture I choose to adopt. Each piece—a small upholstered chair, metal bed frame, burgundy rug, Victorian couch—are placed to create something of a reflection of my spirit. They form a portrait of someone coming together herself, a young woman with a love of history, community, and beauty, with just a dash of rebellion. A rather *large* dash.

Sidewalk Sale

Early morning. 60 degrees. Overcast. Twin Peaks rise overhead for anyone who bothers to look up as Elizabeth and I navigate the hills in her old VW bug, heading toward unknown treasures. The cool air carries us. This is why I came here—for the coolness of Saturday mornings and to find further adventures, even if that meant hunting down a single unchipped side plate at a yard sale when I was not fully awake. But along with that came an unwieldy group of compadres for Sunday brunches, skinny-dipping in the Russian River, documentary films that drew huge crowds at the stunning Castro Theatre, and a fascination with Harvey Milk, our somewhat timid yet amusing photo shop owner/councilperson.

Palm trees fan out their lacy limbs as we climb the hills and descend into valleys—streets lined with Victorians, each a miniature dollhouse brought to life. Pink, purple, pale yellow, many with fancy molding, wide porches, and secret gardens behind. They lie alongside each other like a bracelet, each one a bead, all joining together in a way that craved attention and adoration.

Elizabeth followed me to San Francisco a few years after we met as neighbors in Tucson. Both originally midwesterners, we climb one steep hill situated between our abodes. Dolores Park is our shared view, with J Church streetcars slicing through the side of the park closest to us, the clank of each train reminding us, even though we are far from ground level, that we are city bound. In the rain, the green cars race home.

Elizabeth (the smarter of the two of us) has an Ivy League sophistication and short, crisp style. She works at a big publishing company downtown in the Financial District. She assures me that her car is up for the excursion. "I just took it to my trusty mechanic," she says, while pushing a long strand of red hair from her forehead. Funny, uptight, fearless. I am more disheveled but calm, someone who took a huge leap from the nest, never believing that I belonged in that predictable progression I witnessed back in Milwaukee: born, wed, babies, die. Now, walking up to another painted lady, both of us are excited to see what is inside. Oversized jacket, terra-cotta plant container, a lavender crystal.

Two midwesterners adrift in a sea of Californians. It is true that people here came from elsewhere, but I didn't know many from our part of the country. We know cold. Here, there were only lunch box-sized heaters attached to bedroom walls, like pay phones. No basements, no furnaces. At night the fog rolled over us, like thin white blankets. Being situated between Castro and the Mission afforded us more sun than other neighborhoods, and to make the most of that, we gleefully took to our rooftops and planted tiny gardens out back. This, too, improved our carefree dispositions.

We explored the city together. Elizabeth's well-crafted words, immaculate apartment, and precise rules for living versus my impulsive decisions and ready-for-anything attitude. We went to a Jerry Jeff Walker concert at the Great American Music Hall. He reminded us of Tucson—honky-tonks, boots, Stetsons. That's how it was. In the '70s, this California town is more about disco clubs, men with pierced nipples, and double espressos.

This day, garage sales call, but first comes Just Desserts. Our neighborhood landmark features a dozen kinds of cheesecake, along with extraordinary carrot cake and the plumpest chocolate-filled croissants, cookies, and coffee drinks in the city, all right down my street. "Let's get a treat," I say, and the two of us abandon our transportation for a refueling of a different kind. Elizabeth nods. "It's not too crowded yet," she says, glancing at her watch. We get our lattes to go and a bag of goodies, and up the hills we trudge, looking for loot.

Midmorning. 64 degrees. Some sun. The boys in the Castro have on white tees with red hankies in their back pockets signaling preferred sexual positions. We girls blend in with them like tulips and roses—both just right for a garden, each a beauty on their own. Together, a nice eclectic mix. Pick one.

Sarah has sunglasses as big as the moon, long brown hair with curls that cascade down her back, a V-neck cotton shirt without a collar, enormous hoop earrings, and a brilliant smile.

Neal inhabits a tank top, jeans belted firmly at his thin waist, muscles prominently displayed in his right arm, which is firmly planted on his lover's back. Neal leans closer to him, his head of short hair bent forward and slightly down exposing the white of his neck.

Kim's crop top reaches just above her middle with loose-fitting pants beneath. The sleeveless shirt matches the bottom black-on-black ensemble. Long straight hair completes this simple yet arresting look.

The uniform: blue jeans with white T-shirts. In the '70s, gay men gravitated toward a guy-next-door look. Even in the annual Pride Parade, where just about anything was fair game, drag queens were few. Of course, they performed in many bars, but the majority of men in my neighborhood, with the exception of the discreet but revealing kerchief in their pockets, could be mistaken for any student, or blue- or white-collar worker, and indeed it's because they were. Always a nod or hello for me, even though I began as a stranger in their midst. Little did I know then that I'd survive so many of them.

The neighborhood is bursting with young gay men, most who have just come out. Translation: the Elephant Walk bar, the Café Flore, Orphan Andy's Restaurant, and other such institutions are loaded with attractive men, all hot to meet each other. They mingle doing Saturday errands: a trip to the cheese shop on Twenty-Fourth Street, an ice cream at Bud's, or a stop at Cliff's variety store on Castro. Laundromats brim with customers (no doubt checking each other out amid piles of sweaty flannel shirts, stained jeans, and all those sheets used repeatedly in the pursuit of sex), while commerce of the day occurs casually at bookstores, bathhouses, and boutiques. We girls attack the sidewalk sales of residents whose predecessors were hippies, flower children, bohemians, and beatniks.

Elizabeth spots a navy oriental rug just as the fuel of caffeine and chocolate combine to send both of us into orbit. "It's a keeper," she says and doesn't freak at the asking price. The rug is rolled neatly and the two of us hoist it into the car. So far, so good.

Noon. 66 degrees. Windy. Gray. Crowds form inside Old Gold, a massive vintage clothing shop, and at the Zuni Café, filled with its generous portions of cactus and succulents. More streets to view, household items spread across driveways and front stoops or on blankets. No grass here like in the Midwest. The Victorians and apartment buildings almost touching with little greenery out front. Perhaps a small tree among all that cement and pockets of lawns and gardens out of view.

Our vehicle zips up tremendous heights and down into crevices all in search of an address or the sight of a good pair of used corduroys and a cobalt vase. "Look at this chair. I think it would look great in my room." At age twenty-three, just about everything looks salvageable, useful, and just plain cool. "I could spray-paint this wicker chair," I suggest. Later, I did.

Saturdays in the neighborhood, Castro and Noe Valley, were our favorite. Buckets of fresh flowers, gleaming ripe fruit at outdoor stands, and revelry among the masses—students like me, waiters, artists, and political types—all out on errands. Each weekend held the promise of being great. People independently strolled and yet, as a whole, formed a mosaic of energy and style—California 1978.

Streetcars rolled past, old women toted grocery bags, and young men walked hand in hand toward Orphan Andy's for breakfast, their jeans and T-shirts making them appear to be an entire city of twins. The air felt crisp, smiling faces nodded or greeted each other—gay men to gay men, straight women to straight women, lesbian to lesbian—until it, like the city, became all shook up and everyone shared the greeting. I think the straight men were sleeping in. While the backseat of our car became stacked with purchases, the caffeine wore thin and the morning's promise began to fade.

Midafternoon. Still 66 degrees. Wind calms. Anticipation of fog that evening. Miles of Victorians—pink, blue, yellow. Clouds pass. The radio plays a popular song. We both turn to the windows, singing with abandon the lyrics we know by heart: "I've got all my life to live and I've got all my love to give; I will survive."

Giggling, giving the song all we've got, I wave to a man on the street, a bemused expression on his face. Soon evening will come.

Phil

———

Love found me in the face of one blond and boyish man named Philip, until the day he collected his paintbrushes, canvases, and the gourmet chocolate chip cookies I gave him and headed back to New York.

I don't remember how I met Phil. Maybe it was at volleyball in Dolores Park? From the park, you could see a small building with a sign that read "The Real Good Karma Café." We never went in there, didn't want to test our luck. Somehow, Phil and I came to know each other. He knew all of my other friends and worked as an artist and carpenter. Places to buy good wine in the neighborhood were nearby, along with the best place on earth to drink it and see the skyline. It was in Diamond Heights. There, high above the city, was a succulent garden with a bench facing the twinkling skyline below. Phil, our friend Tim, and I used to go up there to play guitar, drink, and sing folk songs.

For at least six months each year, Phil painted canvases of various sizes with abstract compositions. I fell for him hard—his blond hair, jokes, and everything else. We made love infrequently, but when we did, it was with fervor. Afterward, he always seemed filled with shame, guilt, or something awful, which made him very quiet and sometimes cold toward me. I fled his apartment in the middle of the night when the room became filled with his anguish.

He'd call loudly after me, so that I wouldn't be running through bushes, alone in the dark to get to my place nearby. Or was it because he felt abandoned? Over time, we learned of each other's pasts and how some of those experiences may have affected our relationship. All of this made for a complex and tender relationship, one that was sadly tinged with shame.

The first time we made love was at the home of his mentor, David Ireland, in the Mission District. Although by this time I knew Phil so well that he felt like my best friend, I finally got up the courage to ask him on a real date. After the movie, we went to David's Victorian, where Phil was house-sitting. David, a conceptual artist, had turned his home into a piece of art as well. We had both attended the opening he held at an Irish pub on Mission Street, where video screens showed the work in progress.

Neon ran along the baseboards, and David left clusters of brooms and piles of concrete balls atop stools. David's house existed as his 3-D canvas, a merging of exhibition and living space. His yellowing varnished walls, complete with leftover wallpaper glue, were the custom of the day. Wide wood flooring marked by occasional furniture accented the high ceilings. A long wood table from his African travels, piles of sheepskins on his bed, and mirrors upon mantels—it was in this womb of art and history that Philip and I became lovers. But we kept it a secret, not telling anyone we knew. Until it was time for him to go.

Transportation

Sometimes I think that I spend my entire life riding on the J Church streetcar. All the mornings going to work when I wait for the streetcars to come, and when they break down I try the subway, and when that breaks down I take a bus. I remember all the times of doing just that—jumping off the electrified streetcar, walking down to the subway terminal, crowding on only to have the door of the train fly open and stay that way, with the automated voice telling us that the train is malfunctioning and will not be going any farther with passengers, so I hoof it up to the street again and hurry to a bus stop, where the vehicles move unencumbered by tracks, long rods, wires, and all such nonsense that keeps them from running free.

Financial District

The streets are cold. I walk along them, repeating my steps each day, as in a labyrinth. Surrounded by a sea of suits, carrying double lattes before the rest of the world discovered them. Commuters rise, the three-story escalators of BART stations lifting them toward daylight. On their skin, the dark tones reflect from subway mosaic tiles, as streetcars and electrified buses dump load upon load of office workers onto Montgomery Street, the main artery of the Financial District, often referred to as the Wall Street of the West.

Now a multitude of legs march in slow motion to the blues notes of a saxophone, cradled by a black musician, his left shoulder against a Market Street wall, the instrument's case filling quickly with quarters, dimes, and dollars. I toss in a coin. The soulful and sensual sounds of his instrument compel me. Aside from this gesture and the few words I contribute, most others stay focused on their lattes and scones, just steps away from their offices.

At the intersections, encoded with invisible cues, streams of people set out diagonally, crossing to the other side, along with other skirts and oxfords making the traditional rounds. Much like a flower petal opening, feet taking the part of tiny ants that push open peonies—back and forth, day after day in the sun. A ballet where all are preoccupied within their own thoughts, yet know where, how, and when to walk in conjunction with all the others. I imitate.

The traffic knows instinctively what to do; it stops for this Esther Williams extravaganza, where pedestrians' arms and legs join and separate on all sides, and through the middle, in unison. Each face straight ahead, arms swinging the *Chronicle* or *Examiner* newspaper at their sides, taking a quick sip, a slight turn, and a bounce. Lights blink from above, briefcases work as metronomes, and the clink and thud of a thousand shoes create the rhythm of this morning in the city, my city, where the elegant and aged facades of the Financial District buildings create a funnel in which we flow.

People arrive from every direction and mode of transport, all driven to arrive on time. With frenetic pacing, which did not exist in my life before now, an ocean of people swells and slowly ebbs as each one disappears behind a heavy door, darts up a 1940s elevator, and anchors to a desk like a bobbing buoy, held tightly for the day's work ahead, tethered safely if not willingly.

My destination, the Transamerica Pyramid, is a familiar landmark. Its sleek, silent design garners instant identification, its torso visible from nearly every location in the city. I arrive, trancelike from the journey, crack a joke with the janitor, jump an elevator to the lowly third floor, and pretend to be invisible as I approach my office, late again, by at least ten minutes, fearing the raised eyebrows of my bosses. It is my rebellious nature that makes it so.

Lunch Protest

At lunchtime, the many small storefronts are busy. Flowers in buckets grace the streets, more coffee, croissants, and the intoxicating aromas from Chinatown nearby pull in both visitors and office workers. Small seafood and Italian eateries stuff themselves between not-so-carefully-concealed sweatshops, a Catholic grade school, a demolition site, and a fountain, at which on most days some kind of group or another will hold a protest, complete with bullhorn chanting, signs, and loud, angry people. It seems with each passing day, a new cause is championed.

Many days while eating my lunch on the front steps of a plaza, I find myself encircled by protesters, held hostage with a peanut butter sandwich in my hand, wondering how to escape back to the office with my growing political knowledge. No, it isn't possible to live in this city without becoming politicized. I am no exception. Soon I, too, will be the one marching, shouting, and pleading with quiet strangers. I experienced an awakening in San Francisco—to a noisy, chaotic, yet loving community filled with many causes—and in the end, I carried that activism forward in my life, long after this community was gone.

Now, when I revisit San Francisco, the voices of protest, which still ring out daily, are a comfort to me. They, with a little mariachi music mixed in, make me feel at home again. I welcome the intensity, chaos, and emotion that drive desire to be so public. When I think about San Francisco, I feel passion. Not only that, but nostalgia for a place where the personal was political, where everyone took a stand and expressed it by wearing it on a shirt, marching for it, singing about it in concerts, acting it out in theater, and displaying it on placards in the windows of those colorful Victorians. The mere thought of San Francisco energizes me because its citizens always made the news of the day their personal business. Soon I learned from them that there was power in collaboration, researching and knowing what we voted on, and deciding what I believed in and how I would demonstrate that in the world.

Chinatown

I'm walking through Chinatown back to the Financial District from lunch. I see the old Chinese men in Portsmouth Square playing the board game of Jok Kay. They hunch over to make a move, while proprietors of produce stands look on. I smell the aroma of ginger, pass a few tourists. As I get closer to the Transamerica Pyramid, I see a Catholic grade school sandwiched in between two structures. Nuns stride out the front door followed by scores of Asian grade school students. Their playful voices carry past a boarded-up vacant lot with graffiti painted on the surrounding fence—"no evictions at the International Hotel."

The air is fresh, my walk leisurely. Because of the heat, one of the doors is open to a nondescript building with covered windows. Inside I see the rows of sewing machines. A sweatshop four blocks from my job. What do the nuns say about this? The women crowd around their chores, sound swirls and whirls like a dancing dragon kite. Take-out food rests in my hand. *What, pray tell, is their fortune?* I wonder as I look in.

My fortune's yet to be determined. Not an insider, nor an outsider, I take it all in—the old men, giddy tourists, children on the sidewalk squealing, women hovered over machines, the attentive shopkeepers, and the smell of ginger. Chinatown becomes my backyard now. All that red and gold of Grant Street leads me here.

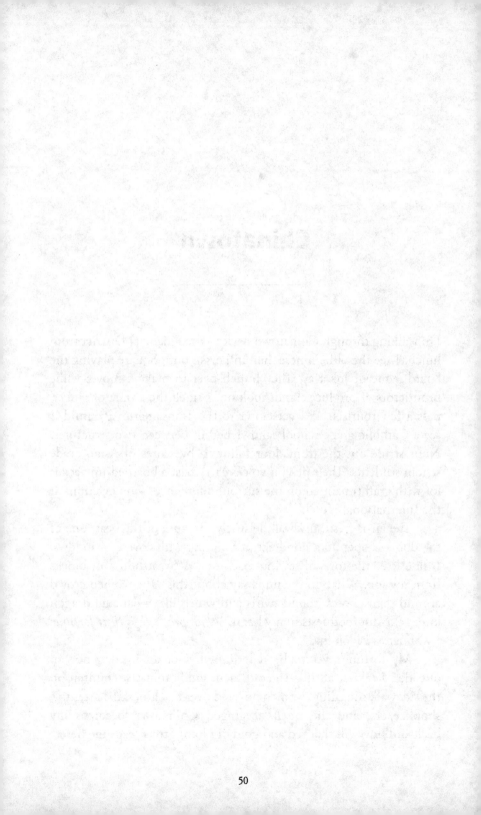

Tim

———

Tim pulls at his bulky gray sweater for a moment, then lifts his head and turns toward me. "Do you want to shoot in here?" he asks, motioning toward his large canvases spread along the middle room walls of his Guerrero Street railroad flat. "Maybe, let me look around a bit," I say, roaming that long hall with all the rooms on the left side. I stop in the dining room, noticing the round oak table, cabinets filled with books. Opposite this room is the kitchen. "Yes, this might be nice." Tim saunters in and I place him at the end of the counter near a narrow mirror, which reveals the room's contents—jars, bottles, and plants.

It also holds his self-portrait. I like to think of Tim's paintings as abstract landscapes. They are certainly big enough to assume landscape status, and the shapes and colors hint at bushes, islands surrounded by bodies of water. Only one other piece I knew of from his collection featured a person—he painted a portrait of his friend Ray with his many birds. Now, here in his kitchen, this self-portrait watches us from the wall, slightly above. The man, balding, sat at a small table with a bottle of gin, tie loosened, looked right through them. I don't intimidate easily, so I take the shot and then move with my camera into his bedroom.

It's hard to remember how or when I met Tim, but we lived next door to each other for a few years. My housemate must have introduced us. Although his passion was painting, during the days Tim worked at a wholesale photography business. We shared that interest and a darkroom in his basement. It drove me crazy that he never cleaned up after his sessions. Consequently, I poured his old chemicals away, cleaned the trays and spools. Only then was I free to start my projects. Aside from this slight annoyance, we were chums. Jumping into his old station wagon, Tim looked like an eccentric middle-aged professor and I the rebellious teen with bell-bottoms, bright eyes, and that curiosity about everything. Off we sailed to an obscure foreign film screening, a photography exhibit, or a bar in some offbeat neighborhood.

I absorbed it all—Tim's fascination with and study of Japanese culture, admiration for antiques, resourcefulness in finding used objects on the street that could be turned into art, like the gymnasium floor he inherited from a friend. He purposefully mixed up the pieces so that the newly arranged floor had patterns, or no pattern, just shapes and letters with no relationship to each other. Another abstract landscape. The floor stunned anyone who walked on it. Tim bought enormous rice paper lanterns and made shoji screens that encased rooms within other rooms. He later lived in less traditional spaces, such as old warehouses and even a Masonic ballroom, and his bathrooms always featured some tribute to Japan—usually a kind of tall metal soaking tub.

When he lived in the ballroom, he kept the largest area with the vaulted ceiling set aside as a painting studio, with only his dead aunt's oriental black lacquer chest and a large paper lantern, called a China ball, off to one side. He lived in a small room in the back and slept in the outer reception room of the once-industrial bathroom. Tim could turn anything into art. He and I ripped surfaces off his walls to see what was under them. We slept on futons and couches dragged into the big room with a dozen french doors open to the bay. We listened to music late into the night and talked—politics mostly. A plan was hatched to move to New York State together someday, get a big house, commute to the city, and be neighbors again. While that plan hasn't come to fruition yet, we still discuss our creative processes in art, poetry, and photography. It's our political leanings to the left that cause us to burn up those long-distance phone lines. Each of us threatens to leave the country for good after various Republican regimes take office, but neither has left, both of us still entrenched in our respective communities.

"Hey, Tim, come in here! Can you make this bed up and sit on the corner of it?" "Sure," he says and with one hand throws the covers across the futon and takes his place in his back bedroom. One of his paintings reveals itself behind him, showing itself to be confident, serene. From the other side, a eucalyptus tree reaches out to touch him. I take my time to set up a bit of mood lighting by creating a shadow effect with the tree, and place an instrument on the side to act as his key light. Two-thirds of Tim's face is in shadow, but one eye and the upper left side of his face remain lit. Despite his comfortable posture—the crumpled shirt and the pant legs crossed lazily on the bed—the position of his head and the sharpness of his left eye leave no doubt that this man knows himself and what he wants.

"Okay, you're done," I say. "That's a keeper." He laughs under his breath and we talk a bit more in the kitchen. "Oh damn," I say, noticing something for the first time that night. "I should have had you take out those paper towels when we shot in the kitchen. They were in the shot." "Oh, so what?" Tim replies. "They're so white, they're going to be distracting," I point out. "Oh well." We spend a few more minutes chatting, catching up. I pick up the paper towels and play with them. He reminds me about that weekend's barbeque and off I go down the front stairs, two feet over, and then up my own stairs to bed.

Tim would become the only gay man I knew in the San Francisco area who would survive the AIDS virus.

Art Opening

Walking up the stairs to the Museum of Modern Art, I try to remember the exhibitor's name. Diebenkorn, isn't it? Yes. That's it. Phil and Tim are painters eager to see the exhibit, and they drag me along. Tim also brings his new roommate, Howie. A physical therapist, Howie became one of the gifts that Tim gave me. He's sweet and we all have a bit too much wine, doing our young best to fit in with the elite art crowd. We're doing fine until I bend down to read a description of one of the art pieces and hear that ominous sound. Yep, I split my pants open in the back. At once my eyes bulge, right hand traces the damage, and panic slides up and out of my mouth. "You guys," I whisper urgently. "Hey! Tim, Howie!" They turn around and silently mouth, "Oh my God!"

Black-clad sophisticates navigate the airy spaces, while Diebenkorn's geometric shapes of blue, lines precisely placed around and inside the blocks of color, provide context to our visit and the room. The visitors roam like insects, back and forth between the paintings, trying to find a new home. "You *guys*! You have to walk in front and behind me so no one sees the split in my pants!" From then on, we move in unison, make a game out of it. Tim in front, Howie in the rear, well, behind my rear in this case. Suddenly I feel like I'm in the chain gang from Woody Allen's film, *Take the Money and Run*. All for one and one for all.

"Hey, let's get some food." We become a column, moving in synchronized tiny steps toward the dessert table. Each of us, standing a little too close to the one in front, giggles. Phil is off looking at the real art. I can't do that at these openings. I prefer to go back later, when there isn't so much distraction. Howie, fresh from New York, where so many people I know are from, is going to go to grad school here. Right now he's got a much more important job being my protector.

Days later, still glowing with amusement from the art exhibit fiasco, I call Howie to reconnect. He had gamely played along that night, following me around, hiding my wardrobe malfunction. He, Tim, and I are very different, but the three of us were united in our mission; we took on that room of chattering sophisticates as though they were invisible and *we* were the only ones really invited. Yes, the art world made us giddy—as we did ourselves, trying to be grown-up.

"Howie's dad died, so he flew back out East," Tim says when answering the phone. The sudden soberness of the news smacks me and puts an end to thoughts of reliving the gaiety of our first meeting. It is so early in our friendship; I don't really know him yet but realize how everything will now change for him.

Ireland 32

A fiddle sings, as if a quick and hungry fox, and a dozen dancers grab hold of my arm, the one resting on the bar. They are taking me hostage, or so it seems from the way they skim and scrape this California floor, all connected like cars on a midnight train in which the locomotive is loose, without a single driver at the controls. This boisterous clan turns to me, a new patron, the bashful woman with the silver streaks in her Irish dark hair, the cow eyes, and flat feet, while the rest of the narrow tavern sings tunes of loss and love, toutin' the Guinness. Dancers of no particular lineage or age slap their circle against the shores of the room, and they make me one of them, knowingly or not, when they pull me in.

Strangers, all of them, except for Michael, crooning into the microphone. He, the friend of a friend, is whom I stay with the first couple of months in the city. He cleans carpets by day and sings of Celtic battles late at night; the Ireland 32 Bar in San Francisco's Mission District is his regular Sunday night gig. The bar was named after Ireland's thirty-two counties, and the interior space glows from within. Just him in this tiny room—he leaves the band at home. Michael sits with the naked mic stand and a few instruments, his deep voice among them. "I've got my hands on the wheel of something that's real, and I feel like I'm goin' home."

We become lovers almost immediately upon my arrival in town.

His awkward lanky body pressed against my naive and smallish frame, my shirt hiding a rash from all the excitement.

I become lovers with that circle of strangers too, who pluck me, alone and hesitant from my bar-side stool, and sweep me into the euphoria of that dance. Going around faster and faster, we make the circle lose any semblance of shape or boundary, and in that joy, we take over the tavern. We become the bar, its identity, its energy, its soul, and its thirty-two Irish counties.

The friends I make in San Francisco become like these steppers; our lives become an elaborate, inebriated dance, which twists and turns in hilarity and high camp, speeding toward some unknown and frenetic crescendo. Although there is a hangover of monumental proportions waiting the next day, the memory of the night before—a night of pure joy, of high and precise kicks and rhythm—carries me like a river. Freedom comes in many forms this night. Coaxed by the seduction of Michael's voice and the tales of forlorn but determined unions, my body becomes fluid, unencumbered by custom or authority. The sheer will of the grabbing and holding by this new community in which I now dwell, one that is alive and nurturing, it lifts me—I am spinning.

I continue to dance each Sunday night, first with the group in one of our instructor's upper flats, where musicians play at our rehearsals. Then we head to the Ireland 32 for a field trip and a chance to try out some new steps in the real world. Once through the door, we abandon our sense of discipline and the regimen of the steps and plow through the wooden floorboards like a brigade of tractors to a potato field. Determined to harvest the most of our evening, we let each step and movement explore the territory of that bar, as if it were Ireland's hills and valleys themselves, each step closer to the mother- and fatherland, each step a joyous toast, a nightcap to our survival.

We dance at fundraisers for the IRA at the Plough and Stars Coffee House, among others. Usually someone from Ireland is temporarily staying with the organizers, sleeping on their couch, an underground railroad bringing these Irish loners, politically too hot to handle, to the States to cool off.

The dancing keeps me moving. Back straight, as if held up by a stubborn yardstick, defiant kicks and turns, and all of our bodies coming together to join arms above our heads to form a star, then moving around it in wonder. The music haunts me. Even though my time with Michael proves brief (he had a girlfriend—a secret he didn't share), we continue a friendship. He moves on to other gigs, while I stick with the dancers and different musicians, with their dulcimers and tin whistles, which tell the stories of my ancestors.

The City

Streetcars roamed the hills and a cool fog rolled in each night. Mark Twain talked about our town. He said that the coldest winter he ever felt was a summer in San Francisco.

I used to love to watch the fog roll in. It wasn't until September that the weather would warm up. By then, we'd be camping in foothills listening to bluegrass concerts under giant parachutes, lying on thick grass. At night, we'd study the stars and crawl like caterpillars back into our down sleeping bags.

Imogen

I kept a picture of local photographer Imogen Cunningham on my bed stand. It's a self-portrait of her from about 1910. A serious young woman, she sits with a tranquil yet determined expression, papers and pen in lap. A soft light plays with her hair, small curls parted down the middle, and her simple dark dress is topped with an enormous square lace collar centered by a cameo. Cunningham lived in San Francisco while I was there. She published a photography book of her contemporaries entitled *After Ninety,* published in 1977, when she herself was that age.

Imogen Cunningham's black-and-white prints of calla lilies and close-ups of magnolia blossoms from the 1920s impress me most. Whether they are singular or in pairs, both the delicacy and strength of these flowers overwhelm me as a viewer. Here, petals swirl into spadix, or fold themselves before the idiosyncrasy of carefully sculptured stamens. These work nicely with the nudes she does of the female form. She entitles one *Triangle,* of a breast, which attracts the geometric shape of light on its timid shape. In a poster I bought in San Francisco called *Two Sisters,* she places a nude frontal view of a woman next to a profile of a second woman. I'm drawn to the symmetry in the women's bodies, their faces and heads obscured. The soft curves and angular lines of their torsos blend; shadow and light add to the contours. But a few white scratches mar the right nipple and shoulder blade due to damages incurred in my many moves.

My burgeoning interest in photography led me to Cunningham and I imagined that even after college, I, too, would continue this interest in camera work throughout my life. These images, mainly portraits and flowers, inspire me. Studying her career showed me that a woman could remain artistic, viable, and independent long into old age. I emulated Imogen and her work, capturing many portraits of friends and using her favorite colors—black and white. Much later, I was to appreciate that I had those photos of friends, as I did not know so many of them would soon be leaving us.

Richmond

I'm restless on a Sunday night. My roommate Rosemary and I (yes, we shared the same name) are hanging out in our apartment on Guerrero with nothing much to do. "Let's go out," I suggest, and with that we check our finances (which add up to zilch) and head for the car. "I think we should hit the comedy club, since they don't charge a cover on Sunday night." We drive in the dark over to the little neighborhood tucked into the far side of Golden Gate Park. There's also a bar over there, where you could hear live bluegrass music seven nights a week. We walk into the club. Narrow, the brown tables and chairs scatter about. I spring for a beer, the only one I can afford. We sit down in our Levi's and flannel shirts. I'm prepared for a somewhat generic experience, but I hear people whispering and before I know what's happening, they announce a special guest. Robin Williams walks onto the stage.

He's in town for his high school reunion and when he starts telling jokes, we double over in laughter. His act goes on for hours. It gets pretty obscene—and he's sweating like a pig—but we find him endlessly hilarious. Robin bends over and screams into the mic. He paces, tosses his head back, spits into the crowd line after line, and starts up again like an engine that revs and sputters and finally roars. Tears. We howl, tipping our chairs, for that's all we have to give him.

Hong Kong

We have our favorite restaurants in the neighborhood, and mine is the Hong Kong. It's funky, with cheap food. I eat there at least once a week. Broccoli with tomatoes. Mmmm. Tonight, Paul and I have just finished eating and we're walking through the dozens of tables to pay our check when he says to me in a slightly raised voice, "I told you, I want a divorce!" I take one sideways glance at him and think to myself, "All right, you're on."

"Oh, really?" I reply with a spark of anger. "Well, I do too! I told you I didn't want another baby!" Heads turn our way as the discussion crests several more times. We continue this nonsense through the checkout process, passing folks coming through the red front door as we step out into the street, and keep it going for a good half block down Church Street, until we both collapse in laughter. The next time we're at the Hong Kong, it is a slightly different script, maybe different players, but the same antics.

Howie

Click. Breathe. Howie sits leaning slightly forward, forearms lying across his legs, fingers gently intertwined. A checkered shirt drapes his upper body, the material creases and folds and puckers on its way down his lean frame. It's bright in the center because of the window light, as if something ornately organic is glowing from his interior. The light spreads out from the center of his shirt, burning the buttons, attaching itself to both sleeves, part of a cuff, a left pocket and gently lands on a shoulder. The only other remaining brightness in this photo is the white of Howard's eyes. They stare into mine. So serene, so determined, so centered. Next to his curly head a white candle looms out of frame. Its holder is just as tall, but partially blocked by palm leaves. His jeans look smooth and comfortable. A piece of classical molding from a typical San Francisco flat shows itself; dark walls form the backdrop above and behind. Howie's head is turned to face me, the photographer. The window light splashes across half his face, half of the long nose, half of his full lips, one bushy eyebrow, a chin, and hint of forehead under dark locks. I see just a hint of light in the darkened eye. Howie sits on his bed, although no one can see it; but I remember.

Subject Matter

I wander the back streets of a great city taking somewhat nontraditional photographic shots. No Victorians unless they are in ruins, no skyline shots, cable cars, or famous bridges. I concentrate on the quiet behind-the-scenes areas. If I'm lucky, I freeze a moment filled with a memory and a story. I still climb the Filbert Steps, jog across the Golden Gate, study the Diego Rivera murals, read poetry at City Lights Bookstore, and drink Irish coffees at the Cliff House—all San Francisco landmarks—but I don't shoot them. What interests me are the smaller and less told stories.

I take my place in the classrooms of San Francisco City College and major in photography during the four years that I am present there. Working part time as a word processor in the Transamerica Pyramid building enables me to afford a large apartment overlooking Dolores Park and a lifestyle that includes Irish dancing, many friends, and an increasing interest in politics.

Meanwhile, I practice making my blacks blacker, the colors brighter or muted with soft-focus filters, learn to use a reflector, a set of strobes. I take instruction for shooting long exposures at night and using a polarizer, which will pop clouds out of a sky. I experiment with different films, papers, and camera formats. Aperture, focal length, depth of field are swirling in my brain. I shoot, reshoot until I get it right. Print, reprint, and reprint again until I achieve the desired effect. I climb walls, stand on top of vans, trespass—whatever it takes.

Mission Dolores

I walked a lot when I first arrived. The streets bulged with humanity. I'm thinking of Mission Street now. Long lines in front of ATM machines, billowing wedding dresses in lavish sidewalk windows, and the smell of little Day of the Dead sweet cakes, each hinting at another savoring moment still to come on this earth.

Mission Street stretched out like a parade of lowriders, flat to the ground and constantly in motion. Boom boxes blasted at top volume, while neighborhood folks and tourists juggled their parcels and errands along the mile after mile of commerce. Taquerias opened their doors wide and presented both their plentiful portions and a brief immersion experience of the land south of the border.

Nestled in the Mission District, along with the crowds of Latino children with dark eyes and hair, sat the seventeenth-century Spanish Mission Dolores, a church and grounds, which always remained dear to me.

The old San Francisco de Asis Mission chapel—its Spanish nickname, Arroyo de los Dolores, translates to "creek of sorrow"—is dwarfed by a larger basilica next door. However, the original adobe fortress is fronted by pillars, a trio of windows, massive wooden doors, and a balcony. A simple cross extends from the colonial pitched roof. Beside it on the left resides a garden that features both historical plants from California Indian tribes of the late 1700s and the remains of tribal members and early settlers.

We've made a plan. We'll come here after the big one. I picked the Mission Dolores because it's in the neighborhood and since it has been around since 1776, I think it would withstand even the biggest disruption. It was lucky enough to survive the great 1906 earthquake. Since the 1906 quake, many smaller ones rattled our lives, but because the Bay Area was situated on the San Andreas Fault, many scientists predicted that another very devastating quake was likely in our lifetimes. Everyone agrees. That's where we'll go, the first Sunday after it hits, at noon.

There's been a bit of renovation, earthquake proofing in town, since the last one. The libraries and schools are having some ornamental work removed, the same with the government buildings. That should help. So we put the word out. John and Paul know. Neal. Kim told her Jon, the new boyfriend. I told Elizabeth. Tim said he's in. That's it. When the big one hits, especially if it's impossible to communicate by phone or anything else, we just all regroup at the Mission Dolores. If the church is down, then we'll meet in the courtyard. Got it? Pass it on.

In a few short years, an earthquake struck worldwide, but in places like San Francisco and New York City, it shook us to our core. It wasn't an event of weather, but a pandemic. We all tried so hard to make it to the Mission, but in the end only a few of us did.

Pride

Every year in June, the city celebrated Gay Pride. Like most other places across the United States, this included a march, but because such a large number of gays and lesbians lived here, it was as if the entire city turned out for this event. For those of us who lived in the city: euphoria.

We began the day at a brunch thrown at a friend's place, where, among other things, we had champagne and probably a few drugs to boot. After eggs, toast, whatever, we piled into the back of a pickup truck so we could arrive downtown together.

Mandatory was the Queen Elizabeth wave to the adoring crowds. One holds a hand high, close to the face, very stiff and straight, rotating the entire hand sharply back and forth while smiling the largest smile imaginable. We laughed so hard. Once again, the attire mostly went toward jeans and T-shirts, but there was always a smattering of drag queens dressed to the nines. Our only quest for the day was to enjoy ourselves, together and apart. People partied downtown and on Castro Street. Usually a crowd of 360,000 joined us for the parade. Local politicians attended. Floats of all sizes sponsored by some of the bars blasted disco tunes, which was the music of the day; plenty of men atop danced.

The atmosphere changed and the lightheartedness disappeared, while a politically charged march, centering around issues and rights, replaced it. I witnessed the beginning of the parade one year, which began with five young people, each with signs representing Stalin, Hitler, Idi Amin, a burning KKK cross, and in the center a sign with the picture of Anita Bryant. Ms. Bryant—commercial spokeswoman, singer, and former beauty queen contestant—was widely known for her anti-gay activism. The actress, who had been verbally bashing gays and most likely inspiring more hate crimes than even she could conjure up, was the new motivation for taking to the streets defiantly. These actions signaled a change and the parades thereafter followed in tone. The subsequent marches emphasized human rights, not just a celebration of sexuality. Some people expressed themselves publicly for the very first time. It was exhilarating to see and be part of this.

Most of my friends (save John) were not politically inclined. I found that surprising. While I eagerly attended rallies, marches, speeches, and the like, they stayed back. Actually, most were introverts concerned mainly with living their lives and not analyzing the world around them. My pals and I held elaborate brunches, attended the parades, but before the speeches began they would filter out, heading for home. I had always done things alone, so attending the more traditionally political events after the march felt natural to me.

In the '70s, I knew my role among the crowd was to report. You could say I was imbedded in the heart of the San Francisco gay movement for the purpose of self-knowledge and the mission to spread the word to some of its most shy members, who happened to be my pals. Sometimes they feigned disinterest, but I could see in their eyes that they knew the importance of every statement made on their behalf. Curious about gay politics, since it encompassed everything around me, I made a point to learn as much as I could. That's how I ended up on the cover of the 1978 Gay Freedom Day Official Program.

The lavender cover sports a crowd scene, with me perched conspicuously in the center. It was taken at the previous year's event. There I am, sweater draped over my folded arms, long straight hair, looking intensely serious at those around me while listening to the speaker up front. One of the proclamations inside the program stated, "On June 25, 1978, the lesbians and gay men of San Francisco, the Nation and the World SPEAK OUT in union with women, dispossessed races, poor and working people, and all those, gay and non-gay, who fight with us for the right to lead joyous lives in a just world."

Surrounding me on the program cover were hundreds of men—black men, bearded men, men with shirts opened to their navels, Asian men in corduroy jackets. Men who were hugging, men sporting carefree smiles and leather, Chicano men standing next to lesbian couples, men with curly mop tops and those with receding hairlines, older men, men in sunglasses with big hats or middle-aged with serious expressions—they were all there. I was their comrade, and I knew what they said was important for me to hear because, in the end, this had become my world.

The Stud

Bodies undulate against each other on the dance floor—the hard, sweaty bodies of hundreds of gay men. Loud music punctuates the air, especially "Miss You" by the Rolling Stones. It is 1978, the second coming of the Summer of Love, and I find myself moving effortlessly toward that dance floor, dancing out into that sea of manhood. Not a straight man in sight (although Paul always swears there are a few) in this massive migration of gay masculinity.

At the Stud, everyone is primed, and sexual energy pervades the place. Not just on the dance floor, but in the bathrooms and dark alley nearby. Men ask me to dance, to snort poppers, to talk. This mirrors my relationships with them in the neighborhood— three hundred big brothers: friendly, protective, and provocative, all wanting to play with me and make sure I am having fun.

The caring and attention between these men and I was enthusiastic, reciprocal, and enduring. Later, it included bedside visits, celebrations of their lives at memorials, time spent sorting through their possessions and participating in die-ins on the White House lawn on their behalf.

Pink Room

It's Sunday morning and I'm waking up in the pink room. Pink walls, small room. I wonder if John and Paul are awake yet. My arm reaches over my head and touches the hard surface behind me, while I shift about in this double-sized platform anchored firmly between Paul's bedroom on my left and John's on my right. I stay here when we've been out late, which usually means out dancing at the Stud. Like last night. Oh, I'm tired and hung over.

Someone's up making breakfast—I can hear the clanging of pans. I had better get up. I finally talked them into buying a stool for me to sit on in the kitchen, while watching them cook, so I best go sit on it. Oops, forgot my toothbrush. Bet Paul will let me use his. What was I wearing last night? Oh, there are my jeans. I've been wearing that green shirt for the longest time. It's ripped on the front hem. Maybe I should fix that. Naw. Time to get up, Rose. God, that music was great last night. Jesus, my head is pounding!

Filmmaking

About halfway through my stay in the city, I began making films, which is what sustained me until I completed my photography and journalism studies. Like most filmmakers, I incorporated many of my friends into my work. They're handy, generally work without pay, and are usually enthusiastic. Because I was drawn to realism, my job was to document.

Castro Theatre

With a penchant for foreign films, documentaries, movie classics, and special screenings, the Castro Theatre, a 1920s movie palace built by the Nasser brothers, drew crowds every weekend. The exterior resembled a Mexican cathedral, and under its Art Deco chandelier sat 1,400 patrons all singing "I Left My Heart . . . ," the old Tony Bennett standard, or "If My Friends Could See Me Now" with the organist who played live before the films. All forms of camp ensued in this giant community center/movie house and, in a final tribute, reportedly the ashes of Vito Russo, author and gay film historian, are imbedded within the theater's walls. The theater was granted landmark status in 1977. Being a film freak myself, I attended often and recall standing in a line that wound around the block to see Barbara Kopple's *Harlan County, USA,* and I enjoyed so many other films there and at the Roxie Theater in the Mission District. Located in the heart of the Castro, the theater held forth as an iconic destination and a guaranteed great time for all, including me.

The Arts

I made my way down Castro to pick up flowers, then a little people watching while I ate pizza, and then took a leisurely walk back home toward Dolores Park. I've been in the city for three years. Ballet, opera, theater—what does a working-class girl from Milwaukee know of these? I drank it all in.

A Chorus Line and other big shows entered my life along with Frank Zappa concerts, trips to the Museum of Modern Art, and the sounds of opera singers who frequented the Corner Grocery, a gay bar down my street on Eighteenth.

Christo's gentle white fabric fences, a larger-than-life conceptual art installation, blew down the hills and into the ocean. Thiebaud and Diebenkorn's paintings mimicked our own landscapes, inside and out.

Gino

Tonight is Gino's birthday. He's working all day at the wharf, but we will mark the occasion when he's done. He'll be here soon. His tired, ruddy hands will be here soon. The flat he lives in is roomy, the housemate absent. I spend most of the week here. We will eat crab—the same crab that Gino cracks every day, all day, at the wharf. The bread will be sourdough and the wine will be white. His body (and hands in particular) will smell like fish.

I remember him showering and still smelling of fish afterward, but the strong muscles of his massive arms excited me and when he lifted and carried me to bed, I giggled. Many nights ended like this. One morning he took me to a Sicilian bakery on Mission Street that had hot almond pastries with melting vanilla icing. We sat in the car eating them and I wondered how I could have lived in the city for this long without knowing about them.

We met when I accidentally left my wallet at his house after a party. When I came back to claim it, there was Gino sick in bed. After a few minutes of conversation, he asked if he could call me. I nonchalantly said, "My number's in the book." So it went—bike rides around the city, cooking together, street fairs.

Our romance ended at Coit Tower, a local hot spot for making out. We drove up the hill one night toward the phallic monument above us. After the kissing and hugging commenced, Gino stammered a bit: "I've been seeing someone else." I couldn't see how, since I'd spent so much time with him. I saw him at least four days per week, so the other couple of days obviously belonged to someone else. Stunned and disappointed, I had no choice but to move on.

The Haight

I walked into Buena Vista Park with my friend, dolls in our arms—a man and a woman doll that had yarn for hair—and a bed, which Erica had made for them out of fabric. The camera swung off my shoulder. The embroidery colored their faces and I had taken Erica's photograph while she sat in a rocking chair at our apartment holding them, putting in a few last stitches.

A real man in another state was after Erica. He had beaten her, and that's how she came to stay with us. I took pictures of my new roommate against huge gothic pillars because she had confessed to wanting to be a model. I remember how Erica's black skirt swirled and how later she leaned back against the wall in my apartment, the 1950s flowered wallpaper creating a nice mat around her blond hair and soft-focus face. Erica told me how an art director had liked my prints. She also told me how she had been afraid, didn't have any money, cringed every time the phone rang—thinking her old boyfriend may have found her. During the years that I knew Erica, her fear of this man never left. I imagine the only way she was able to survive was by always being vigilant about protecting her whereabouts and by allowing for the passage of time.

As time progressed, Erica moved on from the modeling idea and started making art. The doll making seemed to settle her, give her a function. These dolls—some in peasant dresses, others in dark suits—came with actual body parts. Individual toes, breasts, elbows and knees that bent. She would sell this colony of little people, complete with long mouths and belly buttons.

After the portraits, we decided to photograph the dolls outside and went to Buena Vista Park. I remember snapping pictures and then walking farther into the park that glaring afternoon, clutching the soft bodies of the dolls and looking for a pleasant background.

I walked down a short embankment and saw a man standing as a lookout, dressed in black leather. Walking toward him, I noticed his motioning for us not to come closer. My eyes swept beyond him and saw dozens of men huddled together in the daylight. "What are they doing?" I wondered. The urgency of his warning finally made an impression. They were having group sex, the whole lot of them! Bodies tight, arms reaching, knees and elbows bending, cocks and nipples both hard. The individual toes tingling. A hum of pleasure rose and drifted up through Buena Vista's trees. Being relatively new to the city in 1976, I hadn't yet been clued in to the particular popularity of this park.

Sometimes when I think of Erica, this is the image that lingers, the startling one. The one of men clustered into a hive, the frenzy of sex out in the open, on a sunny day. Sometimes it's the tiny velvet purse, which she made me shortly afterward. Mostly, it's the pillars. I can still see Erica's face with the black lace of her hat covering it, the way she raised her chin, pretending to be someone she wasn't—carefree, happy, and wealthy. And letting herself believe it long enough to start over.

Come Together

Come together, then apart. Shouts from the middle, fists fly, earrings flash, moans, rubs, thrusts, pulses, fists, swings, moans, bends, licks, and more shouts. Back together, then apart. Back together, then done. Until later tonight, when it all starts again. Rubbing, bouncing, screaming, thrusting. Nipples pierced, muscles working, coming together—ass cheeks flexing, fists flying, tongues licking, cocks swinging. Coming together, coming apart.

Fisting, nipple rings, and poppers. Taking friends to bathhouses after last call. Sylvester and the sounds of disco echo on Eighteenth and Castro. Later, torsos of the anonymous AIDS dead were outlined in chalk in the streets, victims of a viral homicide. Glory holes. The Stud. The Black and Blue Bar. The steady drip of hot candle wax, weathered leather chaps, and studded choke collars with leashes. Bathroom stalls, where men fucked like flying monkeys in front of my eyes, in caves squatted like squadrons, in bars like ants swarming a hill.

Holidays

Winter holidays—Hanukkah, New Year's Eve, and the like—were quiet ones. No snow covered the streets and I remember walking around gazing at Victorians on Christmas Day only to find the streets emptied of people and other signs of life. They actually seemed deserted. I imagined that most people left town to visit relatives elsewhere or were tucked safely within their own personal enclaves, deep within their homes.

Elizabeth, my Tucson crony, and I spent most holidays together. Usually for Christmas or Thanksgiving, far from our families in the Midwest, we would plan a day trip up to Mount Tamalpais. We spent the morning driving. Upon arriving, we'd grab our backpacks and hike, eating the nuts and fruits we'd brought along, and probably talking about the films of the day.

We both were huge film fans. It remains one of our common interests and bonds. And by that I mean foreign films, independents, documentaries—the quintessential art house showings and the kind of films you'd find at the Roxie Theater or the Castro on most weekends. We consumed them like coffee.

We lacked only in money, so contributed our shares to the gas expense along with a homemade dinner in a small-town café on the way back. These holidays, simple though they were, remain my favorites. Being in the outdoors away from the city and all it represented energized me. However, it felt good also to return.

I didn't miss visits home to my family on flights I couldn't afford. I didn't miss gift exchanges, the tree, or carols—the outward signs of Christmas ritual that never changed. We, Elizabeth and I, had stumbled on another expression of how to be a family. And it was sincere. I think of her still whenever Christmas approaches and I wish I could return, once again, to that time in San Francisco when we knew just what to do.

Here, Take One of These!

Let's make mimosas! Her friend at work gave her the white crosses. They all did poppers. Her legs gave way. He talked his mother into helping them. It was too dangerous to visit them up on the ranch. They had guns. Sure, I'll do some. She brought it on the plane. It had a bite to it. The brownies tasted terrible. Haven't you ever done this before? Her heart pounded rapidly. Let's go out in the alley. She rubs some on her gums. We snorted the lines at brunch. He shook his head. She couldn't sleep. They laughed. She stayed up all night painting. Don't open that here. Make that two Dos Equis. I can't believe you did that. She didn't care. Just get on antidepressants. She had a kit in her purse. He passed the joint. Her brother had been an addict. They got the munchies. Here, take one of these pills. How will this make me feel?

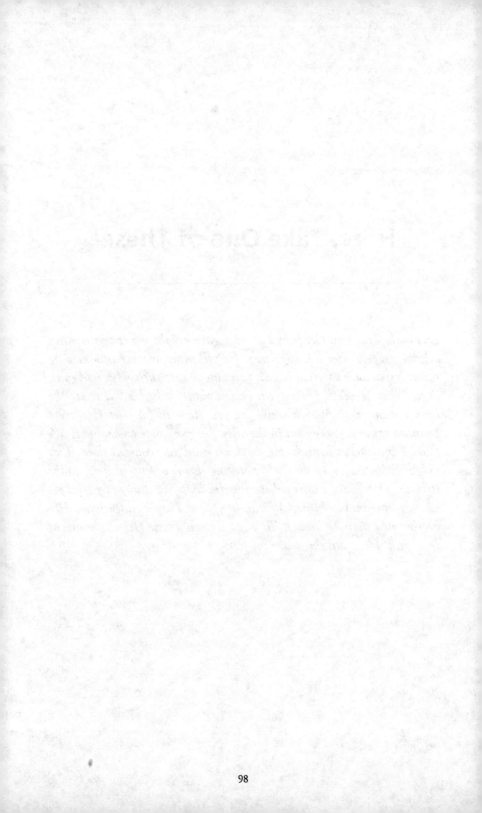

Pamela

My drug-dealing friend Pam, with endless supplies of cash, once offered to buy me a darkroom, but instead, I built one for her. A stranger would never guess her profession and I liked her despite it. Pam posed for my portrait class, and I visited her apartment just up the hill off Castro Street. One night after we sampled the goods, we spent the entire night in her darkroom developing what seemed like hundreds of prints from a concert she went to. The performer: none other than Bob Dylan, born and brought up in my future home—Minnesota.

Pamela

North Beach

I remember walking in North Beach and peeking in windows. You could get countless different kinds of coffee from one of the cafés. Some of the old haunts have always been here, like the waitresses who moved so effortlessly within them. Once, friends and I stopped for dinner at the Caffe Sport, where the restaurant prefers groups and offers large portions, family style, of practically everything on the menu. Each of the many dishes is paraded out by the Sicilian chef and shared by all. I recall how they gave us red wine instead of the white we had ordered and how they called out loudly, "Devis, party of five," instead of Davis, and how everyone laughed and the nickname stuck for decades to come.

After the workday ended, North Beach beckoned. A short distance from the Financial District, its streets were jammed with businesses of every description—Italian restaurants like Little Joe's, Lawrence Ferlinghetti's City Lights Bookstore, curio shops, and strip clubs. One could hear disco from the Dance Your Ass Off Emporium, folk guitar from bakeries, and flamenco, to which strong, sensual bodies stomped in an establishment on Upper Grant Street.

The Savoy Tivoli always made me feel as if I were in Paris. Its main action occurred out on the street, where dozens of tiny tables huddled in front of its windowed front. No matter what time it was, the tables were crowded. Coffees floated past on trays held by sophisticated slim waiters. People sat smoking, reading books, talking. Heaping salads and pastries accompanied the coffees. Sometimes we would sit at the tables looking out. The main activity seemed to be watching people on the street. Very bohemian, like everything in North Beach. Inside, in case the weather was cold, the expanse was larger. But mostly everyone went outside.

The Tosca Café had a waitress who had worked there since the '40s. Her expert hands wiped tables as naturally as if she were washing her face. I watched her once as I strode by the window. Her dark hair expertly curled, black-and-white uniform melding around her supple body. It was her hands, however, that impressed me the most. They scurried across surfaces as if on fire, as if she had memorized the motions, the tables, and their landmarks. She picked up and moved glasses, coffee cups, napkins, silverware in a quiet, measured way that spoke of familiarity, grace, and enduring repetition. She did her magic. Alone, she worked late in the café refilling the creamers. No food was served within those red leather booths. Whenever I think back on the city, she is forefront in my memory. Her name was what—I don't quite recall. Henrietta? Tilda? Doris? Some old-fashioned moniker, just as sturdy as her arms.

Old Hallows' Eve

It's Halloween. This night, more than any other, is for the boys on Castro. I find myself hosting a party and none of my friends, the regulars, are in attendance. Instead, the Church Street apartment is filled with acquaintances I hardly know. I attend as a devil, wearing a black nightgown, red horns, and a sign on my back that says "the devil in Ms. Davis," a takeoff on a recent popular film. I also wear black net stockings. Suffice it to say, I'd never be wearing such a thing back in Milwaukee.

Near the end of the party, a friend and I walk to Castro, passing folks also dressed in strange attire. At the intersection of Eighteenth and Castro, the entire street fills with revelers. Laughter and drinking combine to create a Mardi Gras atmosphere, which makes this a highlight of the season. Rules of normally acceptable behavior seem to disappear. On another such Halloween, my night ends with me kissing a stranger in the bushes of city hall downtown. Hard to remember how that happened exactly. But I remember riding the streetcar home and every person aboard was dressed in costume.

This was also a night when people from outside the city came in to stir up trouble. Hate crimes began to litter our urban landscape.

Halloween became the perfect time to drive up to the city and attack someone gay. My friends John and Paul were beaten one holiday. The attack sobered me, and I realized this violence was a more common occurrence than I wanted to believe. Although my pals brushed it off, it really alarmed me that they had black eyes and bloody noses. I knew it could have been worse but was unprepared to deal with it when it became really personal. None of us were safe. I was beginning to understand that. Harvey Milk knew it too.

One year, I went with my roommate Casey down to Castro and we were dressed as little girls. We put my hair into pigtails and Casey then twisted on old coat hanger, threaded it into my hair through the rubber bands, and then braided my hair around it. At completion, we could maneuver the braids straight up or out, and with the addition of handmade freckles and a too-small dress, the outfit was finished.

Unfortunately for us though, the night we picked to masquerade was the wrong one. It was the day before Halloween. We ran along buses on Castro, being silly, the only ones dressed up. Waving to everyone we saw, we darted in and out of traffic, probably giving an out-and-out preview to many. Indeed, the night would soon be upon us.

Halloween, the night that gave everyone license to be their wildest, to act without regard, to let imaginations run wild, thankfully came only once a year, but that made it a night worth waiting for, planning for, and when it finally arrived, a night worth reveling in.

The Castro guys came in their usual attire, which was plenty of black leather, some with men in neck or arm harnesses, locked with chains. A few lesbians went bare-chested. Many of the bar windows were wide open with patrons straddling street-level boundaries between in and out. It was one wild party. On upper levels, couples necked in full view of the streets below. Music, disco music, pumped everyone up. Donna Summer was her name; euphoria surrounded and swam through the crowds below. Poppers, alcohol, and the darkness were all anyone needed.

It was as if all of the bars were lifted high above Castro Street and shaken until every patron fell out. But add to this mix neighbors, such as myself, friends, acquaintances, out-of-towners—and with nearly everyone in a costume to conceal their identity. Many a butt was grabbed on Halloween and mine was no exception.

With my devil mask on and in a very crowded environment, I delighted in my anonymity and having men pass me as if sniffing to see if I were one of them or not. Once in a while they would say something seductive in passing. I would not reply, in order to keep the game going and make them keep guessing. By the time they did, I was on my way and they were amused.

―――――

At some point on that particular Halloween, I must have crossed a straight man (this is proof that at least one straight man existed in San Francisco in 1979), for we spent the rest of the evening making out in those city hall bushes. I always wanted to do something political, but this was hardly what I had in mind. Pleasant, though I never saw the young man again.

Back at my apartment, the party was still going strong with the hangers-on who were friends of friends and not anyone I knew that well. I tried several times to kick them out and finally just went to bed. I had work the next day. As much as I liked a good party, here I was: my costume torn and dirtied, the alcohol high wearing off. All I wanted was my home and privacy back.

So much for that. By morning they were gone.

I-Hotel

Near my office in the Transamerica Pyramid was the International Hotel, the site of a grueling eight-year political battle between an absentee landlord with connections to Bangkok and a coalition of housing and labor groups, Asian activists, and students who tried to stop the demolition of a low-income residence hotel, home to mostly elderly Filipino men, or *manongs*.

Paul advised me not to get close because it was too dangerous, so I watched from a distance, listening and reading what I could. Even though I did not participate in the protests, their blueprint loomed large in my mind and surely but subtly affected my political consciousness. The action became like an opera that played throughout my entire time in the city. Police came on horseback in the dark, while thousands of protestors were alerted by phone trees to surround the building on numerous occasions. Everyone knew of it, and my friends and I sympathized with the residents. In such an international city, our circle had widened quite large.

Sheriff Richard Hongisto spent time in jail himself for refusing at first to carry out the I-Hotel evictions. His diary from those days was published in the city's local rag *The Bay Guardian*, a newspaper that filled its pages with notices for comedy clubs, singles ads, and exposés such as this one. I remember reading about the demonstrations and wishing I were brave enough to attend. This action in many ways reminded me of the work by Father Groppi, my hometown priest who led over two hundred consecutive nights of fair housing marches in Milwaukee's segregated North Side in the late 1960s. There, too, I observed.

I photographed the graffiti running along a Financial District wooden fence: NO EVICTIONS AT THE INTERNATIONAL HOTEL. Someone had sprawled the letters about four feet high and running fifty feet or so across the surface, which fronted a vacant lot, bordered by old cement and brick buildings. A lone woman walked by wearing baggy pants, wrapped in a long sweater. She passed a parking meter and the back end of a van. A tall cylinder-shaped chimney stood between some of the buildings. The photo's tones run from the darker, dense look of the older bricks to an entire concrete wall lit by the sun. However, the graffiti says it all. It captures the attention, the imagination. It provides the urgency, the demand for action, the narrative of the times. The fall of the International Hotel was an iconic event in San Francisco during 1977, so unless you were living under a rock, you knew about the trouble in Manilatown.

"The police are on their way now. The police are on their way. Go across the street if you don't want to risk arrest. We want everyone to tighten up now. Security people, go to your positions. We want the crowd to slowly move back to the human barricade," said a young woman into the bullhorn.

Police on horseback approach the I-Hotel in the middle of the night. It's 1977. Phone trees alert the followers and approximately two thousand people witness the end of this long siege. Young Filipinos escort the elders, some clad in their pajamas. People from many camps and ideologies come together that night, including neighborhood and labor groups, gays and lesbians. Common people, everyday people, San Francisco people circled the building holding hands. They sang. Prayed. Young and old.

"I'm afraid you'll have to leave now. You can't come back," says Sheriff Hongisto, armed with a sledgehammer. The police brutality on the chaotic streets is clearly documented in Curtis Choy's documentary *The Fall of the I-Hotel*. Tenants finally agree to leave the building after several attempts by the mounted police to rush the building. Many activists are dragged out. Police finally enter the residence hotel with ladders provided by the fire department, evading the crowds below. A dignified yet frail Mr. Felipe exclaims: "I like to stay here. I don't want to move." The International Hotel is demolished soon after this night, with many of the residents' possessions destroyed or stolen, and an empty hole remained on the site for the next twenty years.

Steady John

John was my one gay friend with the steady pace. He had a couple of cats, a soft green sofa, and large hanging spider plants that, for some reason, were immensely reassuring to me, an insecure young woman forming her identity. My constant moving from body to body, apartment to apartment, served as a counterpoint to the contentment and stability of his life. Neal doted on John, and their rhythm hummed along evenly, while mine took more sharp, short-lived paths. My lovers, for instance, were more frequent and less kind. John's domesticity grounded me. We did our laundry together sometimes, careful not to leave our clothes unattended, in case someone ripped them off while we were out getting a bagel.

John not only directed my student films, he assisted in my photo shoots. He would think nothing of spending an entire Saturday pulling together a nice vegetable salad, with french bread on the side, just so I could create an elaborate set in his living room in which to perch said salad and shoot it numerous times until I thought I'd gotten it right. Then we'd happily eat it, and if I was lucky and we had time, he'd give me a haircut. Later that night we'd go dancing.

We had his mother fooled for a while. She thought I was his girlfriend. I never did understand why John, Paul, and several others I knew hadn't told their parents sooner that they were gay. Did they think their folks would stop loving them? Perhaps they were waiting for the right time. I never had to take a risk like that, didn't have that much at stake. It took a lot of energy for my friends to live this double life, and that frustrated me. Stress. I didn't realize that sometimes things didn't work out. People lied to protect their families and themselves. If told the truth, some families closed their doors, hung up the phone, walked away. They lived estranged from one another when secrets were ultimately revealed.

City Lights

It's dark now. I come into the bookstore quietly and head for the poetry section. This suffices, for now. After some time, the motion leads outdoors. I place myself at the vortex—directly in front of the alley, wedged between squad cars . . . could they be part of the act? Looking above, the performer gingerly walks across the expanse of nightfall. He perches daringly on a wire between the City Lights facade and that of the sister building butting up to it. Revelers gawk at the unfolding act; I try to make sense of it, but am impressed nonetheless. I attend alone, witnessing one of many performance art pieces. In this city, they present themselves anywhere—raw, sensual, or like this one, with whimsy.

Neal

Click. Click. Breathe. Neal was hard to catch in a photograph because he was always moving. The few snaps I have of him show him holding or hugging someone. Not surprising. He was so warm, personable, and good-natured that he almost disappears in our group. Like a warm breeze, his presence wafted gently across our bodies. We wanted him to stay close by. Everyone loved him.

At an art fair, he cuddles with John. With Paul, he banters and gets into discussions. He carries baby Cindy, the daughter of our Hong Kong roommate, Serena. And worships Kim, as most everyone does, for she is both goddess and earth mother to us all. Neal finds his way to nurture Cindy on our trips to the bowling alley and Serena when we deliver her to the airport for another visit to China. And me. He's a fabulous listener, and like me, he loves to talk. What could be better? You could say he is the soul of our group.

His tall, slender physique embodies the hopes of a young East Coast guy with dreams of sexual expression. In our John, Neal finds a respite, a solid base. Their domesticity, animals and plants included, offer me a restful and safe place. Neal is strong yet tender. Working in the restaurant business suits him. Crowded tables, with people our own age, clamor for his attention. He gives it graciously, paying attention to the details. People remember his name, his smile. With his friends, he delivers affection, not in a showy way, but with a constant everyday naturalness that defines him.

Conversation with Paul #1

"I hate my job, Paul." Looking around the small Market Street restaurant, I settle on this singular thought.

"Get another one," he says matter-of-factly, as though it were that easy. I pick at my food, scan the familiar surroundings. Wood paneling, short stools, burgers. We spot another friend. Say hello. More nibbling at a meal.

"And I feel really depressed." This said with a frown, a lowering of my head. A confession, a defeat.

"So get on antidepressants. You'll be fine." Paul is earnest, if not impatient. He's done it. He's been there. He knows me.

"Really, it's that simple," he said.

The Earth Moves Under Our Feet

When an earthquake hit (and many did during the years I lived in the Bay Area), there was no time to prepare, let alone react. You maybe had a second to brace yourself in a doorway, or just watch as everything around you shook—plates, tables, light fixtures, beds. Once, late at night reading in bed, I saw the sentences start to tango and momentarily looked under my bed to see what was shaking it. Another time I sat in amazement with six other people in a kitchen. We were stopped mid-conversation and could do nothing but sit in our places as the quake rocked us. Our only clue was a low growling sound, like that of a train. Then it hit.

A fairly large quake struck one morning at work after my company had moved from the Transamerica Pyramid to a ten-story building in the suburbs of Walnut Creek. It was probably in the seven-point range, and when it sprang I didn't even have time to duck under my desk. From our tenth-floor location I saw the outside walls of the building start to roll. Very unsettling and frightening. A coworker stuck in the doorway held on. His expression filled with fright.

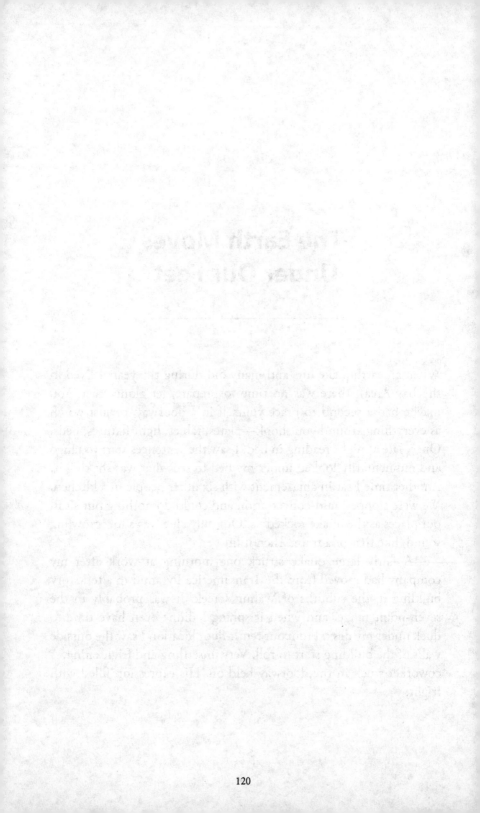

The Apartment

I greet Kim as I come into the Sanchez Street apartment. It's railroad style. A tunnel shoots out from the small nucleus of a living room, the one with the brick fireplace, the red vinyl airplane seats that fit nicely under the rounded windows and black window shades. About two-thirds of the way down the hall is a small guest room. In it is a tiny floral-covered chair for a small-framed person, perhaps one of us. Kim leads me past this room and the alcove, which holds the phone and beyond that double bathrooms. They made them that way in Victorians, a sink and tub in one and the toilet in the other.

Eventually the tunnel opens into the kitchen. This is where the owners must have modernized the old place. It's an odd shape, this room—straight, sharp edges, angular really—and beyond this is the main bedroom with its woodwork crawling three-quarters up the walls, the bay at the end with the three windows, bare except for the deep red shades.

I slept on the floor in this flat once, after I had a falling-out with Leon, who promised to come here from Minneapolis and move in with me. He changed his mind at the last minute. My closets had been cleared, one of my jobs left behind—all for a man who never arrived. The floor felt hard, my disappointment fitful. I would spend several nights in this flat.

About a year later, I moved to the Twin Cities and in with him, but the night when I told Kim I was moving to Minneapolis, she protested. "You can't do that!" she exclaimed. "It's the real world out there." We both laughed, knowing she was right, but I followed Leon anyway.

The Sanchez apartment passed from friend to friend over the years—Mark, Paul, and eventually Kim's sister. I can see the different couches, chairs, and people who occupied it, but somehow it always felt the same, familiar to us insiders. When Paul was sick with AIDS, I'd stay with him here, sleeping on his pristine white sofa in the living room, but hearing the same summer sounds through the front gray-curtained window. I'd fly through the same lobby, skip over the same wooden steps, ring the buzzer with the same secret code, but he would answer.

As a beginning filmmaker, I used the flat for a location of one of my films. Witnessing John and Paul move from one apartment to another, I got caught up in their feelings of sadness and nostalgia leaving the old place. Since their move was already completed, I decided to use Kim's new Sanchez apartment, which was empty, to re-create the guys' move.

I got all the props ready—beer for the party scene, boxes for moving, a plant. I was waiting for the guys to be ready and took an impulsive shot of a neighbor woman in her window two floors down. This spontaneous choice made me feel less encumbered by the script. My goal was to capture on film the feelings of remembrance and sentiment when moving out of one's home.

As time goes on, I continue to visit the apartment. The door is cracked open for me just a bit after Kim buzzes me in. I push it open wondering when the others will arrive. "Hey," I exclaim, taking one look at Kim standing against the fireplace in that tiny worn living room. "What's going on?" I ask. "Rad! Glad you're here early," she says, calling me by the nickname my initials form, and leads me down the tight hallway. "Wow, the new paint job looks great." While passing the bathrooms, I glance up and admire the two-tone gray walls with a slight band of molding painted a sharp turquoise. "Did you do it yourself?" "Yeah." Once in the kitchen, we pause. "How are you, girl?" Kim says, opening the fridge. "Help me come up with something to make for dinner."

We stand in the kitchen, her kitchen, the two of us poised, sharing the trivial chatter of two longtime friends. Behind me, as I sit at the broad wood table, and facing Kim, the deep red shades of the master bedroom beat against the bay windows.

Miss Beverly

The apartment on Sanchez had many visitors. Once when I was there, one of Kim's neighbors stopped over. Ronnie (aka Bev or Miss Beverly) worked as a cook at the Balcony and the Badlands bars. Later, he partied at the clubs. Originally from a small town in Georgia, Ronnie, with his round moon face and gap-toothed smile, could transform the attire he was wearing from Castro Street "regular guy" to "Bev" in no time. With a vast wardrobe of dresses, shoes, and wigs, he often held a fashion show in Kim's apartment before going out. Glitter! Heels, jewelry. Plenty of white crosses kept him going through the long work shifts and into showtime. I'd sit there in the kitchen, mesmerized like the Catholic schoolgirl I was, and ask all kinds of questions: "They did WHAT on top of the pool table?" "When do you have time to sleep?" "What did you wear?"

Kim recalls Ronnie as a softy and a sweetheart. For years, she and Paul would quote several Miss Beverly lines—so many things out of Bev's mouth were instant classics. One came from an incident Bev was relating from the night before, of orally pleasuring a young man in public. They were barely concealed in the back of a truck parked at Sanchez and Sixteenth. A passerby stopped and tried to investigate what was going on in there. Beverly stopped what she was doing and with hand on hip drawled, "Dew yew miind? Ahm just TRYin' to give a decent BLOW job!" Paul and Kim could have each other in hysterics just by saying "Do you mind?" with Bev's inflection.

Alex

_____

I met a man once in a film-changing room on campus. We accidentally entered the phone booth-sized room at the same moment. While loading our rolls of film in the dark, he with his sheet film, I with 2¼ inch, we talked of the busyness of our lives—jobs and schoolwork. It was comforting to know that others were juggling their responsibilities just as I was, with no time for dating. Although we never actually saw each other during the few intimate moments we shared, because the room was completely dark to protect the film, I remembered his voice and caught up with him again later. He was short with dark hair, an upperclassman. Alex passionately took to photography and for a while also to me, as we dated for quite some time.

Conversation with Paul #2

"Paul, you see this tooth back here?" I say, gesturing as we walk down Sanchez Street near my flat. The weather is overcast and we chat as we walk.

"Yeah."

"I had it fixed at the dentist yesterday."

"Good. I'm glad you did that. The one on the upper right looks better too."

I stop in the middle of the sidewalk and turn toward him. "Hey, how'd you know about that one?"

"I just do," he says quietly.

Paul is always meticulous about his appearance, and since we see each other so often, he would notice my imperfect teeth.

I look at him bemused, and my face scrunches reflecting the gray sky. I'm surprised, but delighted.

Divine

"No, I've never seen a John Waters film," I say. "Then we *have* to go," says Paul. "It's *Female Trouble,* about feminists. This is your kind of movie." From what I've heard, his films are outrageous. "Are you sure?" "Come *on.*" It's late, but a group of us pile into the car and head to a theater somewhere about halfway down Market Street near the Civic Center.

It's dark in here. The seats are sticky. Yuck. I'm not sure about this place. I settle in for my inaugural experience with the divine Divine. Mesmerized, I sink into the crummy seat next to Paul, laughing and trying to figure out the story line, while totally grossed out yet compelled to watch this low-budget Baltimore romp.

The outrageous wigs, makeup, and outfits keep me howling, along with the parallels of feminist rhetoric with which I live my life. I have to admit that John Waters has one hell of an imagination, and as a group we convulse in laughter. One interesting tidbit about the film is that the look of Dawn, the main character, was modeled after a Diane Arbus photo of a young family in New York. Her career kept popping up into my life. It's true: life imitates art and vice versa.

Don't know if I'm ready for this kind of high camp, but I'm here. I'm so tired and probably had a few beers, so I don't even commit to memory most of the film. Like many new experiences,

I absorb this one for later consumption. I'm not sure who's doing what to whom in this theater, but tucked between my guys I'm safe. Watching the images on screen, I feel like I'm watching a foreign film, and know only part of the language. I laugh, and hold my breath at some of the raunchy moments, then laugh again. What a strange world this is. Divine is so over the top, he/she *is* the top!

S/he Had Sex

He had sex with a different man every night. She never saw him again. *I* gave you the clap. He told him he wanted to be monogamous. They read to each other in bed. He called it "hide the salami." She went for stretches of time without sex. Do that again—*please, Daddy!* They fucked in the bathroom stalls with the doors open. It frightened her. I followed him up to the roof. Her roommate was a lesbian. He touched her in front of the other men. She moaned. They wore leather. The flame came very close. He was a psychology major. I ran home. The infection was serious so they went to the hospital. Shut up and kiss me! His nipples were pierced. The women at the street fair took their shirts off. I sat on his lap in a bar. Don't touch me. Can you stay? That's an IUD. They wouldn't let her in. He was sitting naked, with a candle in his hand, when I got home. They loved to talk about sex the next day. Is he gay? The two women were instantly drawn to each other. He was with more than one man. I leaned back on the sink and spread my legs. The wax dripped down. He slept with the same man for seven years. Are you hungry? She had sex with strangers the night before every holiday. He flirted with everyone. I seduced the man next door. They stopped talking to each other for a long time. Her nipples grew long and hard. He was from New York and taught her many things. She stayed with each of them for three nights. They were strictly platonic roommates. I came. He kissed him. He picked her up and pushed her back against the wall. Her roommate let him in. How could his dick stay hard when he was so drunk? She painted her bedroom white on white. He was from Minnesota. Are you still awake? I dropped them off at the bathhouse after the bars closed. They had anal sex until she bled. The dildo was passed around as a joke. I talked about sex with my therapist that next morning. They jogged in Dolores Park at midnight. He wanted to be loved. The doctor gave her a shot. I don't know why they broke up. Something really disturbed him. She never came on to me. I knew he slept with my old boyfriend, but he didn't know that I knew, and I didn't know that he was still sleeping with the girlfriend I thought was long gone. She swallowed his cum. He and his lover held hands. *Are you okay?* She read to him in bed. He laughed. That *really* turns me on. She made out in the bushes. I was horny. He never found a partner. I felt isolated. The two men were lovers for twenty years. Asian men attracted him. He spanked her hard. She met him in a bookstore. No, it's not one of *those* bookstores. He put his arm around the other man's shoulders and pulled him close. They checked each other out. He listened. She knew she did not want to be alone.

Conversation with Paul #3

"Paul?" I say sheepishly, leaning against the kitchen wall in his apartment. This is one of our more intimate conversations.

"Yep."

"You know, I'm really kind of afraid of men."

"I know. Get over it!" he says.

David's House

On this night, with beds full of sheepskins filling David's Mission abode, Phil and I chatted until 3 a.m., both afraid to initiate something further. Finally, I said, "Stop talking. Kiss me." So he did. It took me such a long time to get my clothes off that Phil teased me about it for years. The tennis shoes took the longest. I felt very comfortable though. The early morning sex proved sweet. However, we still kept it a secret.

John and Paul comforted me when he left years later. No more rocks thrown at my upper window, no more singing and playing guitar in the succulent garden with the wide view of the city skyline up in Diamond Heights. No more gentle lovemaking in his apartment before I would run home in the dark.

"Rose! Are you still here?" he would call after me. There were times when I stayed. Other times, my feelings drove me out that door and running home past the dark clusters of bushes, dim streets, and empty landscape. Perhaps my past made it difficult for me to relate to straight men and more natural for me to attach so completely to gay men. I would be safe. There would be no sexual contact, or so I thought at the time.

In September of 1989, a photograph of David's upstairs hall, the same hall that Phil and I passed through in our middle-of-the-night romp, made the cover of the magazine *Art in America*. I was visiting San Francisco then, bought the publication, ripped off the cover, framed it, and in my living room it resides, a souvenir from more innocent times. In the late '90s, David became a yearlong artist-in-residence at the Walker Art Center in Minneapolis, where we connected again. More recently, my friend Elizabeth, whose career leapfrogged from reporter to publishing to politics to film promotion to event coordinator to writers' publicist to Oakland Museum public relations specialist, sent me a retrospective they did on David Ireland's work. Again, I renewed my love of art, the Bay Area, and the blond-haired boy/man named Philip. The one who threw rocks at my window and yelled for me to come down and play.

Much later, after David's amazing career and death from dementia, his Mission District Victorian became a permanent museum with revolving exhibits of his many works of art. Paying my fifteen dollars to visit, I followed the docents and other patrons through all the rooms until I finally walked into the bedroom on the second floor. Its simple bed and accessories lay nearly identical to when I was last there, decades earlier. Art, indeed, on many levels.

Elizabeth

Swish. Breathe. Elizabeth rises out of the photographic fixer bath. You can't really see her red hair in this black-and-white print, but I know it's there. Under her long tresses and behind a troubled expression is a smoldering sexual awakening, which takes several more years to fully emerge. Now, still questioning and searching, she works as an editor. Elizabeth sits at her dining room table reading in her uniform—jeans, buttoned-up shirt, and cardigan sweater. The ever-present coffee cup rests nearby. Around her lie her favorite things: plants, books, and an antique bowl full of pinecones. This photograph is a gentle rendering of a complicated woman. She is reserved, scholarly, opinionated, and a perfectionist. I've known Elizabeth since we were neighbors in Tucson, a brief stop I made after Milwaukee. I take many photos of her.

Our friendship endures. She arrived in San Francisco a few years after I did, but we shared the city, as we had with Tucson. Although our personalities were quite different, our experiences were similar: we both were on our own (still are) and had come from the Midwest looking for adventure. We both loved film, books, good food, and being part of communities. In Tucson, our group of friends was wide. In the Bay Area, it took some time to make connections and not everyone stayed. Elizabeth both met and socialized with many of my pals. She paved the way in Arizona, but I paved the way here. It was clear from the beginning that our friendship had power, humor, and compassion. As she tells me now, "You're stuck with me to the end of our lives." Although my place in the world is far less established than hers, I still worry about her. We're both vulnerable. She has the more impressive résumé, but more stress. Mine has more serendipity, less drive. Elizabeth possesses more confidence in herself. We both become quieter when the other is unemployed. We cheer each other on, when not frustrated with each other's faults. And while Elizabeth's sexual orientation is broader than mine, I learn from her what that means. We have no pretenses. I know about her lovers, at least some. She's met some of mine. We discussed sexual abuse experienced decades ago. She knows about my struggles with photography and writing. We can expound and grow angry about politics. In San Francisco, this combination leads to a lasting friendship.

Say It Isn't So

As much as Paul and I were into psychology and endless analysis of emotions and feelings, we decided not to analyze what happened between us after several years of being friends. We went through a period when we became very attached to each other in a romantically sensual way. I never stopped believing he was a gay man. That was a certainty. But we held hands, put our heads in each other's laps, did a bit of exploring with our hands. I could tell that our friends were wondering what the hell was going on by the strange looks on their faces when they saw us. We didn't know ourselves. No one said anything. We contented ourselves to just be with this uncharted intimacy for a while (about a year, as I recall) and then we went back to being just friends again.

Unthinkable

Amid the chaos of an impromptu press conference, a somber Diane Feinstein let the world know. As head of the Board of Supervisors, she was responsible for revealing the news; our duty was to respond. "Mayor Moscone and Supervisor Harvey Milk have been shot and killed." "Jesus Christ!" "No!" could be heard amid the bedlam that ensued in the newsroom during the announcement. I was standing at the copy machine in my Transamerica office when I heard it on the radio. Simultaneously, a coworker ran into the room yelling the facts. Most folks in the building were out to lunch. I just stood there, stunned, trying to take it in.

Later, while cameras swung wildly on the city hall steps, reporters yelled above the pandemonium and pleaded for quiet, a repeated prayer to end the outrage and restore order so Supervisor Feinstein could complete her statement. When she did, the reeling public was left reeling. My response was to take to the streets.

March

We take our places on Castro Street, arriving after quick phone calls and murmured plans. Word spreads about the murders from street to street, office to office, house to house. Within hours of the slayings, we assemble. Composed mostly of gay men, this unofficial memorial march includes colleagues, friends, and members of Harvey Milk's district—50,000 strong.

Tonight, the mood is shock. There is nothing to say. No words. No sound. I am numb, like the others. No emotion, not yet. The swiftness and finality of the murders has yet to sink in. All I can muster is to show up, to be there. I remember the absolute silence. We are simply present.

In many ways, San Francisco was a small town, only eight miles wide. We young people felt like we owned the city and there were certain things in which we had faith—our leaders, for one. We believed that each night we'd go to bed and in the morning, they'd still be there. Not anymore. These murders took away our confidence and hopefulness. We became grown-ups overnight. I felt the natural disbelief of a person in her twenties, but uncommon was the emotion shown by the experienced police lieutenants, seasoned city officials, and longtime politicians reflecting the horror that day. No one could look away; we all felt it.

Surrounded by what seemed like every gay man and woman in

the city, I join the procession because I have been held and nurtured by the community in which I stand. They accept me and, like other times in San Francisco, I'm not judged. The air is motionless as we wait, each in our own private thoughts, each of us pulling away from our daily routine and caked with denial. Even though Milk had prepared a taped message in case of assassination, we, his constituents, never believed this act would come. Now Castro Street grows dark in his honor, for this is where his political career took place.

The autumn coolness permeates our streets and we walk. Clad in jeans and T-shirts, denim jackets, some men with handkerchiefs in the appropriate back pockets—with all of these things in order, we walk. Baseball caps turned backward, sweatshirts, backpacks and skinny asses, muscled arms, and short haircuts, we move as one. I am home, as I have been all along, greeted, befriended, and protected by those near me now, the ones who also call this neighborhood home.

The only things we bring with us are candles. My hand holds one tiny flicker among many. Trails of light accompany me, that and our silence, save the sound of muffled footsteps. My friends and I walk in anonymity with the others, on behalf of the two who, on this night, become martyrs. Gay men dominate the march, as they supported the slain Harvey Milk, but women—neighbors, friends, and lesbians—join the men. Too stunned for any sensible response, together we crowd the streets, our streets, and move solemnly and bewildered toward Market Street. History comes with us.

We gain momentum as we turn onto Market Street. Lesbians with purple armbands marshal us past motorists, the dark trees, the large windows of a Scandinavian restaurant, Harvey's photo shop, Safeway Foods, the U.S. Mint. We travel down neighborhood streets, through intersections, past apartment buildings, flower stalls, hamburger joints, bars, porn shops, and banks. We move like the hours of a long, slow day, thousands of us, drawn to our town's interior.

Streetcar tracks lie slick beside the tightly wound crowds. They run alongside us, while the occasional glow from street lamps and the far-reaching range of our candles' light fall gently over them. The tracks themselves, witness to decades of San Francisco history, fan throughout the city as they did every night, carrying an electrifying energy, a pulse of sorts, which originates downtown with its business district skyscrapers, into Chinatown, then North Beach spindling outward toward larger neighborhoods, past the Mission, Embarcadero, Folsom, Potrero Hill, the Presidio, and beyond.

Each light shines as a beacon, pinpointing our location. Tiny stars drop into a somber sky, all aglow. Moving slightly within their own rhythm and together reaching toward infinity, the lights dance—each different, each holy. Each light resting in the palms of mourners, who grab hold of them, as if clutching to life itself.

Time is irrelevant tonight. Candles hold us, mark us, and unite our dark shadows. In my mind images float by of Harvey in a convertible waving to exuberant crowds, and of Moscone making an appearance at a voting booth. I am numb.

Through the busy intersection of Van Ness and Market, the crowds surge forward until at last we arrive at the expanse of the city hall grounds. People are crying among us. I can feel the emotion welling up in me. I keep a frantic eye on John, so we are not separated. I can't lose him. Here, now, we comfort each other, staying close, speaking without words, our body language communicating what needs to be said. John puts his arm around me and the others stay close as well.

Finally, we are motionless. We arrive. Candles are lifted high in the air by the crowds when the program begins. There is talk in the press that riots will occur tonight, but our community only suffers this night, only sobs. Anger does not find a place in our midst. Bewilderment, maybe. Disbelief, yes. But not anger. Anyone who truly knew us could predict that. We could not harm anyone this night, for the harm had been done to us.

Strong women guide us. Music begins. Joan Baez sings "Amazing Grace," and the sound and strength of her voice sustains us. Holly Near, from the women's music scene, is also here. There are others. Sally Gearhart, who shared the stage with Harvey during many rallies, stands before us again. Campaign workers, activists, and the rest huddle together while Diane Feinstein lets out her raw emotion in the safe arms of our inclusive embrace.

We were so young, and so hurting. Although our nights had

been filled with much frivolity, Harvey stood for so much of what we wanted. More than any politician before, he was symbolic of social change—people power. Up until the moment of his and Moscone's deaths, we took them both for granted. Now we stood in the cold, real streets of our city and realized what we had lost. At least we were beginning to. Great leaders are difficult to replace, and helplessness pervaded the city. I could feel it physically as I strode through downtown streets after work. The winter was dreary, and the rain kept us damp and cold, matching the unsettled and forlorn mood we continued to find ourselves in.

What would become of us? It seemed as if the city would not recover. For months, depression hung over each normal activity, each resident, each conversation matching the gray winter skies. A popular columnist with the *Examiner* newspaper responded to the occasion with this sentiment. He quoted former Mayor John Rolph, whose words line the state capitol's dome, "Oh glorious city of our hearts that hast been tried and not found wanting. Go thou with like spirit to make the future thine."

Rotunda

The bodies were laid out in the rotunda within forty-eight hours of the murders, on November 29, 1978, where I visited them after work. After a private service, the public was allowed to view the coffins starting at 4 p.m. From my job in the Transamerica Pyramid, I made my usual trek down Montgomery, through the Financial District. A Muni bus dropped me close to the Civic Center. I noticed the sky was a bit ominous. Some rain, perhaps. Within the cavernous walls of the city hall rotunda lay the closed caskets. I remained in the long line, awaiting my turn. The formality and grandeur of the location added to the gravity of the loss.

There I found a grand wide staircase lined with hundreds of floral arrangements from across the country, as well as from local groups and individuals. A large red oriental carpet lay beneath the coffins, revealing the only true color in the expansive room. Elegant white candles in gold holders towered over the policeman, fireman, and sheriff who stood at attention and formed Harvey Milk's honor guard. Graceful palm trees resided behind, while the intricate stone floor, enormous in its breadth, was lighted by bright chandeliers.

When my turn came, I signed the book, strode past the bodies, leaned beyond the velvet rope, pausing to say my good-byes. Sobering business this was, and I carried the sadness with me through the exit and back onto the streets. I had come alone and felt that aloneness acutely as I walked pensively down Market Street searching for the J Church streetcar to carry me home.

It took me many years to feel the full impact of the deaths I witnessed in San Francisco. Although the memorial march for Harvey Milk and George Moscone has been repeated every year since the night of the murders, I only attended one—the first.

Obviously, it stays fresh in my memory. Like the ramifications of posttraumatic stress, the events feel as if they occurred very recently. When thinking of them, I relive them. Most San Franciscans would probably say the same.

The news of the deaths of Harvey Milk and George Moscone moved simultaneously through the region, shaking everyone into stillness. They rendered most of the city's constituents into shock and depression, but motivated others into action to fight even harder for the principles in which we believed. The repercussions were widespread, terrifying, and unpredictable, not just in the Bay Area but throughout the country. Harvey Milk, the first openly gay public official, was a role model, mentor, and symbol of hope to so many who were fighting for political change and human rights. His ruthless murder stunned us. Who would believe that such a thing could happen—and that it could happen here, in probably the most tolerant city in America? We got used to the many earthquakes. Some major, many minor. Perhaps the vibrations of substantial political and social change set our town ablaze. Nonetheless, the deaths of these fine men stopped us cold.

Christmas Eve

An airport shuttle bus routinely dropped travelers at a terminal in the Tenderloin, one of the most dangerous neighborhoods in the city. When my oldest brother, Tom, came to visit for Christmas, I decided to meet his plane. I jumped a J Church streetcar downtown, then walked up to the terminal where I caught the shuttle. Along with the addicts and homeless and mentally ill people seen along the route, there were a number of pimps. They were easy to spot in their flamboyant clothes, and they usually said things to me as I passed them. The Tenderloin stance I developed was very simple. My posture straightened; my face toughened. My pace quickened and the no-nonsense aura I projected protected me. I looked directly into the eyes of a pimp and gave him a stare that said, "You touch me and you're dead." It worked and I never had any trouble there.

For having never before left the city limits of Milwaukee, my brother did pretty well on his first plane trip outside the motherland. I think that both he and John feared each other. But after meeting, everything seemed fine. I'm sure their expectations (macho guy meets gay man) were far worse than the reality of two young men meeting and talking. We cooked and shopped. I took Tom to Fisherman's Wharf, where we toured a ship. I think I even took him to an outdoor concert. My brother never told me what he thought of the trip, but he seemed happy. His outgoing nature and midwestern charm embraced my friends.

At the end of Tom's visit, I had a potluck dinner. Tom worked as a cook back in Milwaukee, and he decided on making lobster and a ham. John brought chicken cacciatore. Everyone came—Elizabeth, Sarah, Tim, Howard, and the others. The Christmas tree looked grand next to the burgundy painted walls. People draped themselves over the antique sofa, stood inside the bay windows looking out on Dolores Park, and mingled with drinks in hand while standing on the oriental rug.

After we ate, I stepped away for a moment and when I returned, the living room stood empty. I didn't hear a sound. Then, walking through the french doors into my bedroom, I saw them. All twenty-five of them, like passengers on a raft, sitting in my bed with the rounded metal frame. All perched together, completely engrossed in *The Nutcracker* ballet being broadcast on a small black-and-white television in the corner of the room.

No one moved. One woman chewed on a fingernail. Some were cross-legged, while others wrapped their arms around raised knees. Each was a singular presence within the whole. They were my group. My group of closest friends, who didn't know they were mesmerizing me. Who didn't know that I cherished them at this moment. Who didn't know that it was the strength of art that was holding us together now. Art and community. I didn't see any of the ballet that Christmas Eve. I stood quietly and observed my friends watching it, realizing the significance of the moment for me, a loner, to have so many dear to me in such an intimate display. On this night, it was pure, sweet, and innocent. When the ballet was over, half of the group went to Midnight Mass and the other half went to a gay bar. My brother went with John to the bar, while I happily stayed home and went to sleep.

Rush Hour

I slipped unnoticed onto the crowded walkway, my salt-and-pepper hair flung against the tennis racket protruding from my backpack. Ranks of Financial District workers maneuvered up Montgomery Street like long lines of ants. We strode toward the hub. Feet in heels, Birkenstocks, tennis shoes, and oxfords tracked, while the bustling intersection hummed before us. Market Street was where everything collided in a kind of cascade of sound, motion, and cacophony. Umbrellas leaned forward, along with my lone tennis racket. I readjusted the weight of my backpack.

Rain accompanied us today—all January, really. I tried to think of it as snow. Not because I missed Milwaukee, but because the rain was so dreary and it was wintertime. The showers muted the landscape, human and otherwise. We all tended to be damp, cold to the touch, moods slightly off. When the light turned green, I crossed with the rest—yuppies, the iconic Brown sisters (identical twins in their fifties, with the beehive hairdos), and that crazy woman who thought she was Jesus. I saw her naked on several occasions screaming, "*I am Jesus Christ!*" People walked right by, never changing their expressions. I stopped and stared, thinking this would never happen in Milwaukee, just as a young guy took off his suit jacket and wrapped it around the woman until the police came.

The next day, the woman was back on that corner. Naked again. She, a blip in a busy person's day—a boulder in mine.

The tiny coffee shops closed for the day, rolled down their metal grates until tomorrow morning's espressos made their debuts. Now they stood idle and empty; people rushed past with the same urgency they had this morning, when they were dying for caffeine, perhaps a bit of chocolate, a scone. At the streetcar stop, crowds surged when the trolleys sauntered up. Once aboard, I stood like most and hung on with one arm to the steel railing above me. I enjoyed watching the faces. Other streetcars glided past and I studied the people: the ones standing and staring back at me, the ones lucky enough to get a seat, the Muni drivers dressed in green boxy uniforms, the office workers in their suits and pastel-colored shirts. This was California after all, the street punks with their spiky hair, the old Hispanic women from the Mission whose dark eyes glanced back at me, and look, there was someone with a little dog in a box.

I found myself wedged between two men. One rubbed himself on my leg all the way down Market Street. I stopped breathing. I never saw his face in the crush of people. Almost there. I simply could not move and was frightened by this strange man touching me. Here comes the U.S. Mint, out of the tunnel now, we made that big wide turn and chugged up the hill. I saw Dolores Park—wet, shiny with slick green benches, graffiti on the wall. I yanked myself away. The birds knew. They circled overhead, while I made for the door. "This is my stop," I said. "Let me out." Stepping into my own neighborhood, I sighed with relief from the unwanted advances.

The Gift

Phil and I shut the door and entered without turning on the lights. His mouth pressed into mine. We spun around his apartment in the dark—darkness in the rooms and out the windows, where bushes sat still and waiting. His right arm pulled my sweater up while I unzipped his jeans, my fingers trembling. Our bodies twisted with urgency as our lips hungered for pleasure and passion.

"I shouldn't be doing this," he whispered. "My old girlfriend is coming to visit from New York tomorrow." With those words, we lunged into bed and forgot all sense of respect or obligation to whatever her name was. It was just Phil and I. Again. In his bed this time, within the rooms I had memorized. These walls he had stripped of wallpaper and set in a clear varnish resembled something ancient you'd see in Europe.

Writhing and flipping across the bed within this gilded nest left us dripping wet and breathless. We had been tossed into a blazing inferno, flames leaping from our bodies, climbing the walls, scorching the windows, and causing the radiators to boil from the heat of our passion.

"Oh, oh . . . oh my God. Oh my God. Oh, Phil."

My nails left narrow crevices in his skin, and I breathed deeply while hearing some music from his upstairs neighbors and the sound of his creaking mattress springs. "Are you okay?" "Yeah," I said. I tasted the wine again in his mouth and noticed shadows in the room. My legs clung to his back and we rocked, slowly at first, until each motion brought a sense of euphoria—back and forth, dark to light and back again—while our tongues played jump rope. He was possessed; both of us used our hands to outline the other's torso and adrenaline took over and we drove around and around, like a runaway train in the dark recesses of those grooved and scratched walls. We rode each bump and valley, each mountain creek and sunny meadow until our desires were sated, then collapsed side by side, exhausted.

The next night, Phil's old girlfriend arrived and left him with a "gift." She unwittingly gave him VD that he then passed on to me and that, in turn, I passed on to a man I met in a bar and never saw again. I called my one-night stand when I started showing symptoms. Another man that I met visiting from New York chose to have sex with me even after I told him I was infected. Where it went from there, I don't know. Probably to the older woman he moved in with shortly after returning to the East Coast. Phil told me the origin of all this six months to a year later, when he finally found out. I didn't understand and couldn't get my head wrapped around the fact that I got this infection from someone I knew so well, and liked. I naively thought I could only get venereal disease from people I didn't know. I wasn't angry at Phil, just stunned. These were strange times, and unbelievably, they were going to become even stranger.

Conversation with Paul #4

"You know, you should wear makeup," Paul says on one of our walks in the neighborhood along the four blocks that separate our apartments. "You really should."

"Grrrrrrrrrrrrrrrrrr, oh come *on*," I moan in my best Gloria Steinem imitation.

"No, really. Dye your hair. Wear some mascara and eyeliner. You'd look really good," he says, glancing my way as we continue walking.

Paul is always after me about this, but I am more into not shaving my legs and armpits, which is the rage these days. I'm a jeans and T-shirt kind of girl. No fuss. Not a girlie-girl. Due to heredity, my hair is turning white, even in my twenties. Wearing makeup makes me feel objectified by men. I like men, but I also like my independence.

"Oh, Paul, let's not start that again. I'm a feminist!"

He looks frustrated. "Okay, so be a feminist who wears lipstick then."

I roll my eyes.

Phil

———

Knocking at door downstairs.
"Casey, will you get that?" *Answers door. Comes upstairs.*
"It's Phil. He wants to talk to you." *I'm not feeling well. In pajamas.*
"I don't want to talk to anyone now. Tell him, okay?" *Casey goes back downstairs. Talks to Phil. Comes back upstairs.*
"He wants to talk to you just for a minute."
"Oh, all right."
I go slowly downstairs. Knocking continues at door. "Rosemary?" *Phil asks.* "It's me."
"What do you want?"
"Can I see you for a minute?"
"No, I don't feel well. Can you come back another time?"
"This will just take a second."
"I can't see anyone right now."
"I have something to give you."
"Oh. Can you just shove it under the door?" "No. Not really."
"Then give it to me later." "Just open the door a little bit."
"Oh, okay." *I open the door a bit. Phil slides a red rose through the crack of the door.*
"Happy Valentine's Day."

Oh God of Life

One January, I exchanged good-night nods and shared smiles with people in Victorian row houses on my way home. As I passed their welcoming porches and dormant gardens, I realized I was being followed. It was dark. Earlier, I had noticed a man staring straight ahead into an empty intersection, his eyes fixed on nothing. This seemed rather odd, so I crossed the street and sped up my pace for several blocks.

Soon, footsteps close behind signaled a warning, but the nauseous feeling in my stomach told me it was too late. Feeling the stranger's hand tightly gripping my upper arm and his menacing presence behind me, I slowly turned and faced the barrel of a large gun.

I sit upright at an interfaith service at the National Cathedral in Washington, DC.

"Just do as I say and you won't get hurt," the perpetrator blurted. His gun aimed at my skull said otherwise. All the pretty houses had fences that kept me from getting inside them. Those many folks I had just acknowledged along the street and on those porches had vanished.

Three hundred choral singers invoke the healing powers of ritual.

Hysteria ran through me like a jolt. The struggle was no longer just between the assailant and me. More overwhelmingly, it became a conflict within me to resist the increasing panic. My body shook violently inside my long wool coat.

I pray as the clergy begin to minister.

"You're okay, you're okay," I recited aloud, over and over, as a mantra. Passing just a few blocks from my apartment, we headed toward Dolores Park. I kept forgetting to breathe and soon the whimpering began. In desperation, I commanded myself to think of a plan, while my eyes rapidly scanned the landscape for any possible escape routes. I found none.

"Touch with your healing power the hearts of all . . .

"Please don't hurt me," I pleaded through my tears as we strode quickly toward the darkness ahead. I forced myself to visualize him raping me and tried to reconcile that image with my future. Yes, I could survive it, but what if he shot me afterward? Suddenly, I realized that I had a choice here. The answer: an emphatic NO!

"all who are burdened by anguish . . .

With this decision firmly grasped, fear instantly slipped past me like a clearing fog, while my adrenaline-fueled body readied itself. I waited. The night felt eerily still; crisp air surrounded us. I glanced back; the gun was no longer pointed at my back but alongside it. Energy exploded within me, my mind sharp. The time for action was now.

"all burdened by despair . . .

With one stunning turn, I seized the momentum of surprise to steal that gun with my eager hands, yanking it as hard as I could until it sprang free. Hidden deep in someone's driveway, we tangled in a wild brawl amid my scattered college homework. I faced him fully for the first time—a young man with trembling shoulders, a carpetbag to hold his weapon, and a yarmulke upon his head. Staring into his blank yet determined eyes, an understanding transpired— no compromise, no mercy.

"all burdened by isolation . . .

Retaking possession of the gun from my now-bloodied wrists and hands, he took on the stance of a murderer. He steadied his stiffening arm, bent his knees slightly, then extended and cast his weapon directly toward my crouching torso, trapped by a garage and thick hedges. I felt desperation, until I reached inward for my voice.

162

"and set them free in love. Hear us . . .

At that defining moment, my piercing scream sent dozens of sleepy San Franciscans scampering to their windows, where they found their voices to order the man away. One man rushed out of his house, down the porch steps, across the front yard, and through the fenced gate to bring me back to his home. Inside, light encircled me while I spoke incoherently on the phone with a female cop. I sat in the kitchen panic-stricken, unable to hang up the receiver. Stephen, the young gay man who liberated me, tended to my bleeding hands, sat with me, eventually waving good-bye. The bay window in his Victorian home was crowded with succulents and cactus. I waved back to him.

"O God of life."

Aftermath

The next night on the phone, I told John about the assault, and he insisted on coming over. When I went downstairs to let him in, although it was dark, I could make out that he was holding a plant with white blossoms. I was startled to see them, or any other flower alive in the dead of winter and I paused at the sight of my dear friend and his thoughtfulness. Previously, I'd gone through difficult times on my own, and I didn't really know how to ask for emotional support. At his insistence, John slept on my couch that night, as he had done one other time.

I had asked him to stay over on a previous occasion, because a young woman was found murdered across the street from my apartment on the playground at Mission High School. Taking a shortcut on her way home from one of her part-time jobs, the single mother was raped and then strangled with her own undergarments. I stood in my bay window, looking down toward the playground and shook. Thank God John stayed that first night as well.

I again trembled while telling him about my experience with the man and his gun. Having John in my apartment made me feel safer, and I was finally able to sleep.

Leon

———

Climbing the stairs after my commute home on the J Church, I shifted my purse a few inches higher on my left shoulder. It was dusk, but I could already sense the slowing of my pace as I neared my apartment door. I entered into the hallway with its exotic floral wallpaper and what I saw in the living room startled me. Leon, a man I had met a few months earlier when he was visiting from the Midwest, was sitting nude in my living room. He had lit a candle and placed it in my front window. Now he sat before it quietly on the wood floor. I was so taken aback by this sight, but it is part of what drew me in. Leon, with his nontraditional ways, was not afraid of his sensuality. Nor his vulnerability, his creativity, or his intelligence.

At our first meeting, I thought he was gay. He kissed and flirted with every man at the table. As it turned out, he wasn't completely straight. Very few folks were in those days. He and I walked together after dinner. A few minutes alone produced this conversation: "How long will you be in the Bay Area?" I asked. "Just passing through," he said. "I'm just here for tonight." I thought that would be it. But somehow, a spark struck between us that sent both of us traveling to see each other in the coming months. One such visit resulted in the naked candle episode. Consequently, this seduction and intimacy pulled me toward the Midwest. The Twin Cities were not a place I'd ever been before meeting Leon, but they were growing on me with each visit.

In time, we decided to live together in the same city. Complications forced Leon's move out West to evaporate, but within a few months, he asked me to move to Minnesota. After much thought and finding a film school there that I wanted to attend, I said yes. It was time.

Leaving

I leave San Francisco on a winter day. A few weekends beforehand, I drag myself up a familiar hill, the one at a steep 45-degree angle in front of my golden building, lugging a menagerie of belongings. There, on Eighteenth and Church, I deposit my stately upholstered chair, where I once photographed a wine glass for an assignment at City College. A spindled side table of dark oak, which a friend convinced me to sell to her instead of to the antique dealer, who made the rounds that day inquiring several times during my garage sale. A corner bookcase, reddish, with five triangular shelves (which I've always regretted selling) and other treasures too numerous to mention.

I felt rather odd that day, with all of my inside things standing on the outside, as if I myself was likewise exposed to anyone who might stroll or drive by slowly to check out the goods. Upstairs lay the empty nest, the one most cared for of all, and the only one I lived in alone while here, after a long succession of roommates in other places. Amid all these treasured pals and roommates, I had found my own place.

And like Virginia Woolf described in *A Room of One's Own,* my place gave me the opportunity to concentrate on college. I built a darkroom in its walk-in closet and wrote film scripts within its walls. It gave me freedom to create.

The apartment is perfect, and now I am leaving it.

My Place Revisited

I pack my boxes tightly and send them on the train to Minneapolis, where my boyfriend, Leon, retrieves them. The darkroom fits into several large cartons; it goes (and stays in those cartons for the next thirty years, although I never stop photographing). Next, my clothes, artwork, my film school application, and the contents of many collections—photo books, rocks, miniature plastic cows, and robes. I pile the notebooks and syllabuses of four years of photography into a sturdy brown box and with it thoughts of late-night study sessions, Morrie Camhi's passion for teaching portraiture, the romanticism of photographer Edward Weston, my visual explorations of the Warehouse District, and scads of images—real and in my head—along with the first shot I ever printed.

One friend, Sarah, takes my white metal bed and curved dresser to New York City when she leaves. A journalism pal buys the burgundy oriental rug. Elizabeth becomes the owner of a few pretty plates and the last of my plants. Even the apartment goes to a friend, that and the pale flowered couch. For a while when coming back for visits, I stay in my old apartment, which gives me some comfort—the same rooms I know, the same view of the park, the birds circling. In the middle of the night, I know my way to the bathroom, along the wide hall with the retro flowered wallpaper, the crisp off-white trim I painted when Valerie moved in. This makes me smile inside.

My lesbian friend offers me revisiting privileges, until she too moves away to Los Angeles, eventually taking a husband and producing a brood of boys.

I used to find it very disturbing when gay people went straight, or vice versa. It took awhile to understand that between the absolutes were some gray areas. I didn't realize that the lines of sexual orientation are far more fluid, less rigid, than I thought them to be. It wasn't that people I knew were keeping secrets; it was that they didn't even know it themselves, sometimes until they fell in love.

Once I came back to visit San Francisco with Arlana, a lesbian friend from Minneapolis whom I met in film school. We went to an art opening with her friend from the Bay Area and my friend Elizabeth. During the ten minutes or so that we were in the car, sparks flew continuously between Arlana's friend and mine, leading them to an eventual relationship. Elizabeth cut off her long red hair, quit her publishing job, and from that time forward had relationships with women.

I accepted this, but felt confused because I thought I really knew her. So why didn't I know this? Why didn't she tell me? I came to realize that she might not have known herself at that point. She was much happier than she'd ever been and that was obvious in her body language and demeanor. All the same, I felt bad when her heart was broken by this woman.

Eventually, when she declared herself bisexual, I was jolted again, wondering where her desire for men was coming from after all these years, when all she did was criticize them.

Omelets

Everyone is here. Well, almost. John is in the kitchen making omelets. Someone with a camera just snapped a shot of the two of us near the stove. It's Elizabeth, who's having a grand time. So the boys are cooking omelets for the folks who have come to send me to Minnesota. Champagne bottles seem to empty themselves, mixed with orange juice, definitely not the kind that Anita Bryant has advertised. Conversations soar along with disco—Sylvester probably, or Gloria Gaynor—which makes it difficult for me to hear people on the telephone sending good vibes. I can see Tim, my former next-door neighbor from Guerrero Street, along with his old roommate, Howie, who long ago joined the ranks and became my confidant. He moves to the kitchen to help with the omelets. John cooks more than thirty of them, each one a little different. Gifts pile onto the coffee table, laughter spikes the air, and the cavernous burgundy living room becomes crowded with classmates, neighbors, the Stone Soup gang, and more. Connections with old friends are strong, and I carry on communication with fellow Bay Area residents with phone calls, letters, and cards after I move.

For the longest time, San Francisco gave me the freedom to act out all of my fantasies—photographer, political activist, and career woman. I experimented with drugs, lovers, the things that many tried in their twenties during the mid-1970s. When I accepted

Leon's invitation to move to Minneapolis, I had one vision in mind. I saw myself ice skating, even though my mother forbade it when I was a child. On a smooth, serene piece of ice, I saw myself gliding across a snowy outdoor rink, alone but happy.

With a photography and journalism degree in hand from San Francisco City College, I reluctantly say farewell to city and friends, moving to Minneapolis in 1980 with my newfound love, a down-home photographer, Leon. My portfolio of pictures and reels of film leave me with many relics from my San Francisco days. Portraits and movies of many friends, including those who would soon die, accompany me. I consider them a living record. That was my role then, to witness and preserve. It still is.

Bus Depot

The week before I leave town, I revisit my favorite San Francisco haunts in between packing. I gaze at Diego Rivera's fresco for the last time out near the beach, sit in the Japanese Tea Garden where I used to study for exams, cruise the Museum of Modern Art near the Civic Center, and see one last movie at the Castro Theatre.

I climb into Paul's car. Now we are driving to the bus station. "Do you mind if we stop at the store on the corner for a minute?" We stand close to one another inside, no need to talk. I handle each candy bar slowly, as if that alone will postpone the inevitable moment when I will have to leave this exquisite time of my life. I'm aware of what I'm doing and yet the moments remain intimate and tender; Paul and I, picking out our last treats of the day, this day that I will not be able to leave behind.

The station soon looms before us. The two of us hug while the bus engine runs, exhaust from its tailpipe pervades the air, and wrappers from McDonald's blown by the wind obscure the graffiti on the side of the building. Inside and out, there is the stale smell of cigarettes and oil. Paul, the one who decides to give me away, his soft red locks, shining eyes, sarcastic tongue—he says good-bye for the rest.

I sit in a seat halfway back on the Greyhound bound for Oregon, where I'll visit some redwood friends before heading to

Minneapolis. Paul eyes the suitcases of the other passengers; they are stacked, a buckle or strap missing from most, and then they are shoved into the cavities below. I glance at him, trying to smile, waving, wondering if indeed this is the right thing to do—moving away. I know it is, yet the thoughts in my mind are streaked like the glass surface of this Greyhound bus pane; the parking lot debris swirls in the wind past my anticipation.

Then something distracts me toward the front, and when I look back out the window a second later, Paul is gone. A feeling of momentary panic emerges, but I calm myself, thinking, "It's okay. It will all be okay." On that sunny afternoon, I imagine Paul as he returns to his car, pulls his blue jean jacket collar up, and starts the engine. He'll return home, meandering the familiar streets I've come to know and love so well, see the friends I love and have cherished.

The panic returns as I am gripped with the fear of the future, the fear I'm making a grave mistake in leaving my secure and beloved city and world. But the fear is balanced by my conviction that it is time to go—this chapter of my life concluded, the next about to begin. A honk from the bus fades along the highway that is bright with rays, as long as Paul keeps on looking.

The Birds Knew

I was blessedly alone among all these people—the boys from Castro with their short haircuts, the well-groomed yuppies from Noe Valley, the freaks from the Haight in their tie-dyed shirts and shoulder-length locks—I loved them all. The boys gave me a home, a haven from the Financial District job, the ups and downs of school, and the pitfalls of romance. They nurtured and accepted me. When they started disappearing, it was my turn to reciprocate the kindness they had shown me. I returned during many seasons to write obituaries, to watch slides from vacations taken in Thailand projected high on kitchen walls, to dance in the aisles of Safeway Food Store, and finally to shower with petals and praises the memory, the memory of this time, with these people, in this city.

The birds knew all along but wouldn't reveal it, not even to me. The light, the glorious light—it shifted, but none of us noticed.

Grieve

Minneapolis, 1982

After a February storm, snow piles border the roadsides, while icicles dangle precariously from wooden garages, lined up like ducks in a carnival game in the frozen alleys of the Twin Cities of St. Paul and Minneapolis. Folks clad in puffy down coats shuffle along the walks, while a group forms at the postal station next to Global Village, an import shop on the West Bank, a neighborhood defined by its proximity to the Mississippi River and the University of Minnesota. Students gather within the New Riverside Café. The special today is vegetarian pizza, which is what I order before heading to class. That and the rice with veggies become the staple of my diet in this, my new hometown.

The enormous glass windows of the café normally act as the community's bulletin board, sharing news of births, deaths, concerts, and the like. Looking through them, I can see there is a double feature of Fellini films playing at the Cedar Theatre located directly across from where I live. Later, I celebrate my twenty-ninth birthday there, alone, watching the famous *La Strada* and *Juliet of the Spirits* starring Federico's own wife, actress Giulietta Masina—a dream double feature for a film lover like me, which I consider a good omen on my recent arrival. Leon treats. All this I see, under the shadow of the Metrodome, amid the stately Foshay Tower, moist underbrush of the Eloise Butler Wildflower Garden, and the iconic Mary Tyler Moore house.

Heading to St. Paul, an evening in 16 millimeter film editing awaits me. Afterward, the class meets up at Johnny's bar, where the dozen of us partake in what is affectionately called "film therapy," which consists of trying to figure out how we fit into the world and upon what subject we will next turn our cameras.

A beer or two later, I take the 16A bus down University Avenue until I reach the West Bank at about 11 p.m. Looking up from the street, I see the light is still on in the second-floor window of this century-old department store building, meaning Leon is there. I smile as I climb several flights of stairs, juggling the backpack of books ready to burst, somewhat tired but happy, bursting into the six-by-twenty-two-foot rectangle we call home.

Leon, in his bib overalls and beard, greets me with a bear hug, while I stand on my toes to reach up to him. We sit among our sparse furnishings in front of the eggplant-colored fireplace in one of the former offices of the old Holtzermann Department Store, now home to students, artists, and me, not deterred by the tiny lofts carved for us with sheetrock and duct tape. Leon and I swap tales of the day's events like two old buddies who haven't seen each other in years. We probably were better suited as friends than lovers. His childlike positive attitude and nonconforming nature appeal to me, much more than his thoughts on monogamy.

We spend rare moments together in the years we live in that speck of an apartment. Both of us work in the daytime, and I go to film classes four nights a week, plus Saturday afternoons. During these years in the early '80s, we actually share only about three dinners together. I had been searching for something nontraditional in a relationship, but perhaps there was too much freedom in this one and not enough of a foundation. Regardless, we jokingly renew our living together arrangement on a week-to-week basis. My part of the rent is forty dollars a month.

In Minneapolis, especially on the West Bank, some young people remain inspired by the '60s, with their tie-dyed clothes and long hair, while others work or shop at co-ops, fight against greedy landlords, or form their own vigilante groups against rapists. I join one such group. As a feminist, I also join a support group of women in film and video. Through members of this group, I become introduced to an entire new circle of women friends, all lesbian, with whom I remain connected for many years.

In addition, I make friends with our neighbors and Leon's extended pals. This motley crew swirls together across the wooden floor at the Union Bar on Monday nights, where we square dance weekly to Pop Wagner and the Black Label Boys. Later, after AIDs takes hold, I think of square dancing in an entirely new way.

Square Dance

A great square dance begins with the legions of the dying. Grab your partner, bow and swing. Gather on up in one long line. Pick a new partner, cheat or swing. Leave your neighbor, Jim, behind. Circle on up; turn to your corner. Bow and swing. All hands join in the middle and form a star. Circle that star. Now step on back. Grab a new partner, bow and swing. Leave your coworker, George, behind. Approach each other; then step on back. Do-si-do. Bow to your corner. Grab a new partner, bow and swing. Now step forward and form two lines. The first couple, make an arch; the rest of you dancers go right on through. Now split off on the other side. Those on the right, please take your seats. Those remaining, grab a new partner. Bow and swing.

Bring those wheelchairs right on in. Form a circle. Bow to your left. Bow to your right. Lock your arms and swing. Leave a dozen or so behind. Grab a new partner, bow and swing. Now come on out and form two lines. Wheel on forward. Now slide on back. Leave Lenny, your lover, behind. Grab a partner, bow and swing. Stomp your canes; spin your chairs. Pick a new partner, bow and swing. Leave another hundred behind. Turn to your corner. Face that corner. Promenade. Now grab a partner. Bow and swing.

Thanksgiving

For Thanksgiving, my new Minneapolis friends retreat to Northfield for turkey enchiladas, football, and old westerns, hosted by one of the physics professors at St. Olaf. The crowd ventures to Ely, in northern Minnesota, on Presidents' Day weekend for annual ski outings, the highlight being a naked sauna with fifteen people and exhilarating plunges into a frozen lake through a hole cut into the ice. No, this certainly is not San Francisco.

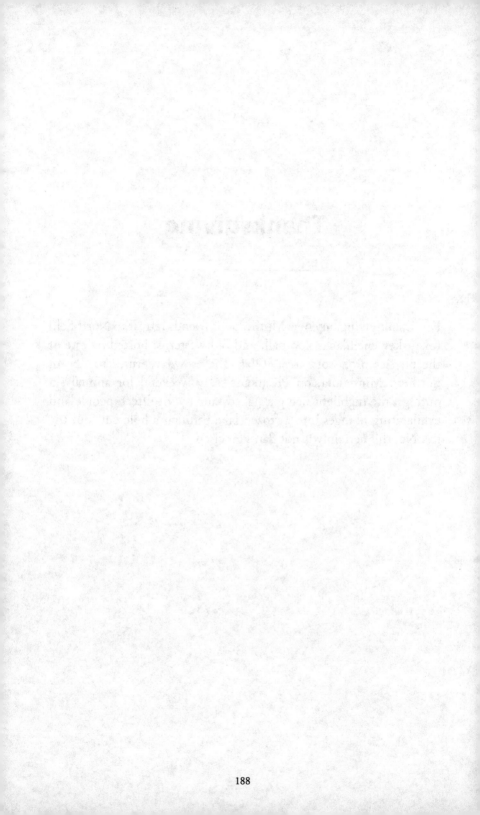

Plunge

In northern Minnesota, I stand next to my friends—naked. In the womblike confines of the tiny sauna, we wait. Warm, dripping sweat, we make small talk. An errant elbow here, a stretched leg there. The wind takes my thoughts, flings them into the sky, and makes a handful of snowflakes out of them. A huddle of torsos stand, so close to the fire. Then, out to take the plunge. One person grabs on to each side of me now; these escorts are responsible for yanking me out, once I dive through that hellish entryway—a casket-shaped hole cut through the frozen lake. The intent is to walk through the dark night from the hot, cozy group sauna to our icy solo jumps into the water. Lanterns on the ice hiss. The whiskey goes down too easily, just as it had down all my ancestors' throats before me. But, I said, no more. Socks, my only comfort, stick to the snow, while the dark skies drop their facades around the edges. Paths, like hot coals, lead us, our skin pink and tender, eyes adjusting to nature. Treading solemnly, we wander along these steaming passageways between sky, water, snow, and ice. Always, we are here to learn, to feel, and to experience. Soon I am in position, looking right down into it. The blackness, bitter cold, standing naked now—even the socks had to go. Taking one last look about, savoring the last drops of whiskey on my tongue, feeling the hands of others awaiting my return, I plunge straight down and in.

My thoughts are wiped clear upon entry and the sensation

is pure and immediate shock to both my body and mind. With unconscious survival instincts engaged, my legs and arms clamber for the edges of the ice in a desperate attempt to escape. My body is jolted by the temperature and intensity of the water. Get out! The others wait around me to help pull me out. With the air temperature warmer than the water, I walk about comfortably outdoors, naked in the snow. After another warming period, I stand in line to take the jump again. This time I think I know what to expect and believe I can handle it. However, once I jump, the experience still knocks me blind.

Moving On

I had been ready to leave San Francisco when I met Leon, and I knew our relationship was the closest I'd found to the intimacy I wanted, even if it wouldn't last.

Life together was a daily adventure. Our relationship endured episodes of drunkenness and Leon's fear of commitment. He wanted an open relationship, but when I tried to connect with other men, he couldn't tolerate it. So much for equality.

After a few years, Leon moved to the Oregon coast and I to a larger apartment in the Holtzermann Building. We have remained friends to this day.

After graduating from Film in the Cities in 1981, I worked on several independent films and later studied video production in which I found a new profession.

I learned to look a tornado in the eye, along with a flood, a raging blizzard, and the farmers' drought. I shared the intimacy of space and time with people who shared their stories. Five thousand interviews. The number daunting, and the experiences enriching.

First Few Years

When I come to know AIDS, I warn my West Coast friends. "Be careful," I tell them, not knowing it is already too late. Denial is very strong in San Francisco, a city built on tolerance and a youthful hedonism. When AIDS shows its face, it is incomprehensible for us to think that we could die from having sex. No way. Could this really be happening?

In the first few years of the epidemic, this is what I hear: talk of a gay cancer somewhere in New York, Houston, and other major cities. Rumors are rampant. Respiratory problems develop quickly. Bacteria or virus, which is it? At the Café Flore, a young man reads the newspaper to a friend. Scores of people come down with the cough. Friends no longer kiss me on the lips. Talk turns to whispers.

Experts say that over one thousand young men died in the Castro neighborhood that first year. I begin a series of visits back to care for sick friends—visits that would continue for another decade. With each trip, a sorrow grows, but also a determination. First strangers, then acquaintances, and finally my closest friends take on this fight for survival against AIDS.

While my friends on the West Coast continue their descent, men I know in the Twin Cities are dying as well. The sheer number in such a concentrated area is what makes the San Francisco AIDS experience so dramatic, but the Twin Cities, like elsewhere, begin to experience a mounting number of deaths.

I join hands with others around the tiny lake at Loring Park in Minneapolis, sharing silence. On Memorial Day, we gather in an old church saved from the wrecking ball by a gay politician, Brian Coyle. The program includes words from a friend of a man with AIDS, a caregiver, a lover, and a family member. Two partners stand, ask the TV cameras to stop filming, and then thank the community for supporting them during their illnesses. They are farmers who have been political activists their entire lives. A bell tolls solemnly as the group leaves the church. The two men who spoke are no longer with us the following year.

Every gay man I've met in these Twin Cities reminds me of those I met in San Francisco. Every man who links his arm with mine walking down a darkened street on a Friday night reminds me of one who came before. Every potluck filled with gourmet dishes made by friends reminds me of food that came before from other friends. Every small apartment filled with roses, white shutters, a blackboard in the kitchen for his friends to write on, and the sounds of waves calling out over bedroom speakers reminds me of other bedrooms painted pink or purple, giant ferns hanging in corners, and other men wearing tight shirts and jeans.

Armageddon

I choke on a spoonful of Cheerios one morning, unexpectedly spotting an obituary in the Minneapolis *Star Tribune* with a name I recognize. Because he was one of the touring managers of the NAMES Project Quilt, his passing is widely shared. The next time I'm in San Francisco, I leave a bouquet of zinnias where Scott used to live in San Francisco. He was from Georgia. We both loved the soundtrack from *The Mission*. I met him when the quilt came to Minnesota's Metrodome. I worked as a volunteer and was in charge of sound for the program and music during the display. Later, Scott sent me postcards from the road as the quilt continued its tour.

After a frantic search, I locate the ex-wife of one of my neighbors. She hasn't heard from Chuck in years. She is still furious about being left by him—for a man. I listen quietly to her rage. Finally, I tell her to bring the children to the hospital *now* because this man will be dead by the end of the day.

In the first few years of the epidemic, this is what I learn: the importance of touch. Of laughter. Of time. I bring roses, truffles, and my overnight bag to the West Coast. I listen, tease, watch slides from their travels. Make promises to care for their roommates, their friends, and their lovers. We cry together. We dance. Most of all, we learn to live in the present. Ultimately, I plant love trees, give eulogies, clean out their apartments. I write an obituary, placing it with a driver's license and other effects in a tin, which is buried in the backyard of our apartment building in Minneapolis. The man's relatives decided against a funeral, so neighbors give him at least this much. The *Bay Area Reporter* becomes one long obituary—he died suddenly . . . his longtime companion . . . he was 31 . . . 27 . . . 42 . . . 35 . . . 24 . . . services pending.

AIDS is an inferno just inside my bedroom window, rat poison in our food. It's a tidal wave slamming into Castro Street from all sides— no letting up, no mercy, no end.

I record sound during the interview of a four-year-old for the television program *Dateline*. Becky suffers from complications of AIDS and is adopted by two gay men (after her addict mother's death and father's disappearance). She loves the huge dollhouse displayed in the lobby of the Methodist church where we gather in Milwaukee. She stands next to me on her tiptoes to see inside the tiny rooms filled with miniature furniture and toy figures. "Daddy, Daddy," she cries, looking for the two men who are now her family, "look at the dollhouse!" That's when I melt. Despite her constant pain, the producers make this child sit through a long interview that they immediately decide not to use. I want to slug them. Months later, I print up copies of her obit and send them to the videographers and other sound people who worked with me that day.

I watch a friend's distant relatives arrive from out of town and ransack his apartment, never asking how he lived or died. They casually discard the hot dinner I give them and go out for fast food.

A colleague hires me to transcribe an interview with an HIV-positive man, Kevin, and his friends from New York City for a Red Cross prevention video. I spend weeks typing alone in a fancy Minneapolis office downtown, learning as I go the most intimate details of this person's life. It is like reading his diary. He tells me how he discovered his first Kaposi's sarcoma lesion. I begin to feel as if I am part of his care group.

Dusk brushes away memory of the day. Stoic young men on Castro Street leave pharmacies clutching shopping bags of adult diapers, prescriptions for AZT and pentamidine inhalers. Humor rises above the street noise. Light shimmies on the wires above, filters down to scorch car roofs, making abstract patterns with tree shadows on the slabs of cement and the reckless and crumbling curbs below. At the laundromat on Seventeenth and Noe Street, a crowd of emaciated figures folds their laundry patiently. All this occurs among the stately palms on Dolores Street, the muddy waters of the Russian River, and the aromas wafting in from Chinatown.

I volunteer at a fundraiser hosted by Minneapolis politician Brian Coyle, held at a mansion he borrows for the occasion. I twist my ankle that night, hurrying across the front lawn to the grand entrance to begin my shift. Vice president of the city council, Brian takes the money donated at his party and divides it among his favorite nonprofits: a health clinic, a theater company, and a Native American youth group. I have to keep his illness private for six months because he is a public figure. Brian finally tells everyone, freeing himself from the stress of secrecy, finding unexpected kindness in the public's response, then dies.

A mutual friend organizes his funeral. An Irish band, hired for his wake, doesn't show up. The funeral itself is difficult for me emotionally. It's held at Wesley Methodist Church, which he once saved from demolition. Native Americans begin the service by blessing those gathered with sweetgrass, the church by now filled beyond capacity. City officials and county commissioners mix with gay activists, ward residents, and campaign workers in the pews. At Brian's request, Senator Paul Wellstone gives the eulogy.

I fan myself with a program and imagine that I am in a Southern church, for the heat is nearly unbearable. The gay chorus sings the local favorite as a finale: "Walk Hand in Hand with Me." The funeral motorcade drives through his district as he instructed, as he would have if he'd been able to run for mayor. For a week, a flag in front of city hall is flown at half-staff.

AIDS is all the leaves dropping from my favorite trees, one by one. It is a damp fog rolling in at night and penetrating nearly every household, a lone drummer beating out a rhythm we can't escape. AIDS is a precise life sentence of two years and three months, no more. It is a great equalizer in a city that used to shine. It is the end of the party.

In San Francisco, my former roommate Casey and her husband, David, care for their coworkers and neighbors. Everyone around them is sick. They buy them groceries, make dinners, and send reports to sets of parents via long-distance phone calls each night. "We can't handle this emotionally," Casey says, leaning toward me. "We may have to move out of the Bay Area."

During a board meeting for an AIDS journal published in Minnesota, the editor unsteadily walks in and sits beside me. His breathing is labored; I hear the fluid gurgling in his lungs. He's missed four meetings in a row due to illness. This time he arrives with passages of brilliance; moments later he's out—nearly unconscious. However, Carlton keeps coming back—that night and for the next months and years until one day when he stops altogether. He is the strongest man I know.

When I start to grieve, the surfaces that hold me while visiting a San Francisco hospital feel as if they are crumbling away. My hands cover my face, tears flow unabashedly. I reach for the walls to steady myself and they assist in the most rudimentary way. I regain my stance to face the death around me.

I finally decide to get tested because of my sexual involvements with bisexual men. Along with two friends, I enter the Red Door Clinic and take a seat in a metal chair against the wall. They do not ask our names, but simply give us a number. When it is called, I go through a door into the back area, where a nurse greets me. When my blood is drawn, I observe it. Will something in these bright splendid drops kill me? The receptionist explains that I must return in person to get the test results. Bring your number, she says. The coming days move very slowly. I can't help but obsess, even though I try to distract myself. When I finally return to the clinic, there are counselors standing by. One young man takes me into a small private room. I sit nervously, looking at his face for a sign, a hint of what is to come. I am negative. With that news I feel immense relief; but the survivor guilt continues because I drove my San Francisco friends to the bathhouses after the bars, where they possibly met their fate. I can't shake that notion from my head.

AIDS is waking up homeless in a wheelchair. It is being at a gathering in a park when storm clouds cover the sun, and the light never returns. AIDS is having a black dress always ready. It is going away and coming back many times. It is lesions, thrush, pneumocystis pneumonia, high fevers, blindness, tuberculosis, and neuropathy. AIDS is turning old overnight.

My neighbor's utilities are shut off. Each morning he goes to his neighbors in his pajamas, borrows the phone, and calls coworkers at the airline. He is too sick to go in, he tells them. They gladly take his hours and he stays home. This goes on for months. His finances draining, he is forced to sell his antique furniture, one piece at a time. I am one of his neighbors.

I sob when introducing myself at a support group for family and friends of people with AIDS. Over the next few years, these people become my family. Each Thursday night, I make the trek to that small reserved room at a Twin Cities hospital, where so much emotion resides. (When I come home, I drink a beer in a darkened room and my housemate Larry comforts me.) We document the progress and pitfalls of our loved ones' conditions along with our own states of mind. Core members leave the support group, one by one, after recounting the deaths that eventually come, until every original member is gone, but me. Finally, I share my own particulars—the black dress, the wake, and the sorrow—with a group of new participants, all traveling the same distance. Then I, too, get up and leave. My time with the group is over.

Day of the Dead altars appear each year now in our homes. Made with marigold flowers, food and drink that the departed would enjoy, and the photographs of those honored, this Mexican custom spreads through California and is adopted in the Twin Cities as well. I ask each former support group member to bring something for an altar at a five-year reunion of the group. Each November 1, near All Souls' Day, we welcome the dead, on this one night, to visit.

During one of my visits out West, Elizabeth cares for three male friends who are dying at the same time and recounts to me how she gives massages, visits, and bathes them. Terrazzo stairs lead to entryways two or three stories high—multicolored, flat, pointed, gated, some covered in graffiti with wild rose bushes draped generously in front of bay windows. I hug her tightly while we're walking down Valencia Street to get a coffee at one of the shops I knew well from my years there. Everyone I know in San Francisco is doing this precise thing. They are either caregiving or they are dying. Or both.

I attend an interfaith service at the National Cathedral in Washington, D.C. Three hundred choral singers invoke the healing powers of ritual. I pray as the clergy begin to minister: "Touch with your healing powers the hearts of all who are burdened by anguish, despair, or isolation, and set them free in love. *Hear us, O God of life.*"

AIDS is raking all the bright green leaves that have fallen into a huge pile. It is a bonfire, ferocious in its size, strength, and heat. It is a forest of stripped boughs. AIDS is a city on fire—stoked with erotic passion, contagious love, and funeral pyres. It is unrelenting.

When we turn to action, some don't understand. I ignore them and get busy. Bleach kits need assembling; condoms need to be dropped at the bars. Marches and wheelchairs up front become the norm and timid fists find the sky, as surely as poets read verse each weekend at City Lights Bookstore, as surely as Muni J Church streetcar bells ring on corners in Noe Valley. Volunteers cook hot meals and a convent is used as a hospice. Walks and rides become fashionable fundraisers. These activities take place throughout the country. I meet an entirely new community of men and women in the Twin Cities. People step forward. Once again a circle forms.

I attend a candlelight march at the reflecting pool in front of the Jefferson Memorial in our nation's capital. The actor Richard Gere brushes past me. Thousands raise hands and lights to the darkness. I do so with my uncle, the closeted one who has worked for the Pentagon all these years. I urge him to join me tonight. He hesitates but at the last minute decides to come, and he spots a group of his coworkers whom he never expected to see here, at this massive rally in Washington.

AIDS is the darkest joke you'll ever hear. It is betrayal, a mushroom cloud descending. AIDS is a sniper with unlimited ammunition high atop a roof: I'll take this one here, and over there, and these. . . . AIDS is a clump of leaves trampled in the gutter. It is despondency, panic, resignation. A god with no mercy.

I stand in a white room during a San Francisco wake and show one of my student films featuring two of the deceased, when I realize that almost all of those standing around me laughing are themselves in various stages of dying of AIDS. I pause, looking at everyone again, only deeper this time, then resume laughing. I laugh because there is nothing else to do. I laugh because they are laughing.

I met Tom on a holiday at his parents' home in New York. Dinner is presented by a maid, which makes me uncomfortable. She brings out blue-and-white china plates manufactured at the family's own factory, so large I am afraid I'll break one. Afterward, I talk with Tom in the den, and we laugh together. He lives in Seattle, works at a gay bar. Our connection is brief, but a bond is made. When he dies, neither of his parents attends his funeral. A suitcase of money is divided among his cousins. One cousin, the one who had brought me to the holiday dinner, gives me a picture of Tom as a young boy. I keep it.

———————

A three-year-old dies this week of AIDS. I met his grandmother in a support group and make her a card with a Celtic design—black and white, four quadrants repeating a pattern of baby animals and fancy borders. The child's mother continues her public speaking and monitoring of her own health.

———————

I sit at the foot of Chuck's bed at a nursing home on Christmas Day. He is curled in a fetal position, thin and wasted. I gaze into the box of holiday gifts dropped off for him by volunteers. He'll never wear those slippers or that robe, since he is too weak now to leave his bed. I read the notes left by friends, sick themselves. He won't be reading these, as he is beyond that now. When a male nurse stops by, Chuck sits up briefly, takes two sips. The nurse yells into his ear, "Do you know who this is?" What's left of the man I know nods his head up, then down, slowly, and utters the only sound I hear from him that day. He says my name.

AIDS is being ignored by society, the government, and your president. It is becoming invisible and being marginalized. AIDS is being shunned and shamed. A black bag of leaves sits on the curb through the night, to be picked up in the morning by a garbage truck. It is abandonment, then finally rage. It is challenging the drug companies, stopping traffic in the Financial District, learning about our own bodies. AIDS is transformation from a victim to a fighter. AIDS is political.

One night I howl in anguish while driving in my cold car. Furious with God, I yell and shout until my face matches the color of the exhaust escaping my vehicle. This man I mourn, Jack Castor, tour manager for the NAMES Project, traveled and set up the AIDS quilt displays. I worked with him, watched him mourn his two lovers.

A close San Francisco friend stops having sex in 1982 when he first learns of AIDS. It doesn't matter. He and everyone he knows dies anyway. He lasts the longest, until 1993. Uneven, cracked squares of cement lie across crumbling Eighteenth Street, from Boyland to Dolores Park. Streetcar tracks bob and weave with the roads, while webs of transit wires tango above. The crisscross of transit wires holds us all in. Sometimes he drinks as a way to escape it. Music helps, humor. He buys me a silver pin and returns all the photographs I've ever taken of him.

One of Elizabeth's friends is moving and I've come along to help. From a second-floor landing, I look out a window into the backyard and at the building behind it. An old tattered sheet hangs loosely in one of windows. "What's that?" I ask. "It's probably a death house," Elizabeth replies. "PWAs go there to die." I stare at the sheeted window, imagining that beyond lay an uninterrupted flow of anonymous gay men with no family or friends to ease their way. In my mind I see them spending their last weeks, hours behind that dirty piece of cloth and wonder how many have left the world this way.

A moonless night settles itself above San Francisco. Restaurants and shops look familiar, but black floral wreaths hang on their doors, this custom adopted from Chinese merchants. Magnolia trees, camellias shed their blossoms, dark moss and burnt leaves cling in clusters to branches sandwiched between telephone poles and street signs, while curios rest in windows of square and round bays nearby. Homemade signs in the windows announce departed employees; advertisements for hospice care abound. Gay bars are empty, and the bathhouses boarded up. All this occurs among the jewel-toned Victorian houses, the serene blueness of the bay, and the vastness of vertical hills.

No sound emits from the night, while the city sleeps. The fog does not lift. Men and their partners, the ones who are left, simmer in sheets wet with anticipation. Funerals are so numerous that people begin to attend in everyday attire—shorts, T-shirts, whatever. The dying is integrated into the routine of living. I find it hard to accept this transition because I am traveling back and forth from my present to my past, back and forth between California and Minnesota. Everything has changed since I left them. I still struggle with denial; sometimes I cannot face the ones I love who can no longer stand on their own. *Forgive me.* At times, I run away, lose control of my bowels before a visit, lose composure on the phone, or forget to call. At times, I am a coward. With each visit, it is as if I am thrown back into hell. All is dark. All is dark.

There came a time in 1988 when the hardest thing for me to do was to walk down the street. Everywhere I looked I saw, heard, and felt death. Friends in San Francisco whispered to me, "It's relentless," "I'm not getting tested," "We didn't want to tell you." So many young men on the streets were emaciated, coughing, carrying canes, while bravely heading up steep hills. The sight defied all logic, until it became the norm.

When those bodies were swept away, so were ones that I once held. Each passing became a separate sorrow that joined with others to create a collective grief—a grief that lone candles, peach-colored roses, handmade signs put up in restaurant windows, unchecked messages on answering machines, and marches into the night couldn't stop.

First Ten Years

In San Francisco, I know that most who worked at the New York City Deli are dead. That apartment building on Sanchez Street, the one where many of my friends once lived, has turned over many times because so many of its tenants have died. The sounds of World Beat music lead a parade down Market Street. I dance to the rhythm while watching the various musicians and groups make their way past me. One of the floats, "The Coming Home Hospice," is topped with young gay men waving to the crowd. Later, I make a hospital visit, only to hear the sounds of men screaming in the background. If they are lucky, their lovers' mothers will comfort them. Sometimes all of this is too much. I need air. I need somewhere to escape, to find a place that lets me express my feelings—to sob, to rant like a mad woman.

He Knew He Was Dying

I am so sorry for your loss. Was he in a lot of pain? He was an IV drug user. She got dementia. They adopted her after her parents died. He was asymptomatic for many years. Did you call his parents? He called in sick to work again. The hospital is letting him out to go to a concert. He needs a ride. Is AZT the answer? He didn't make a will. He lay in his own excrement for days. She did the lecture circuit. They were a family. He told her not to get an abortion. I've got the flight information. Which hospital is he in? I never knew what happened to him. Do both kids have it? She was homeless for many years. He's on a special diet. This doctor is very good. Can I stay with you? His neighbors are dying too. She drank the water. They took everything. I talked to the social workers. She was very angry. He didn't want anyone to know. They went on vacation. I confronted him about his drinking. She worried about her son. He said it didn't matter. They whispered to me what was going on. He lay in a coma. It's time to go now. He took his shirt off and handed it to him, when his dying roommate said he liked it. His brother had a very hard time of it. She stayed in the upstairs bedroom. I'll see if I can get back there in the fall. His leather jacket was stolen. She wrote everything down. The death certificate was so formal. No one went to the bars anymore. He slept with a stuffed animal. She called when she could. Be careful. His sentences didn't make sense. He was so glad to see them.

Double Image

A barn outside the window of my first San Francisco home on Twenty-Ninth Street became the subject of one of my photo assignments. I shot the barn with a pinhole camera directly onto a piece of photographic paper—a paper negative. I was able to print both a positive and negative image of the barn, without the traditional film negative. I mounted them together, twin contrasting barns. They look fundamentally the same with dramatic differences. Because these two photographs were black-and-white, it was easy to see the changes. In the positive image, the barn's roof, houses behind it, and sky were white. But in the reverse image, while the trees in front of the barn shimmered in white, most of the barn, houses, and sky were blackened. Like these images, the city's emotional frame of mind went from white to black almost overnight. The views were virtually the same, but one was colored by sorrow.

The dying stopped me. Stunned me. I couldn't move forward, sometimes still can't. AIDS became my Vietnam, my Holocaust, my September 11. The Castro turned into a death camp and through my visits from Minneapolis, I was let back in. Women friends in San Francisco like Jackie, who even when she was nine months pregnant campaigned for Harvey Milk, leaned forward and whispered, "I didn't want to tell you, but . . ." The stories that followed showed me the strain on everyone there, especially the caregivers. "AIDS is relentless," they said.

Demonstrations organized by the AIDS Coalition to Unleash Power (ACT UP) fill the streets. Whistles shrilly blow as if to scream, "STOP! THIS IS AN EMERGENCY!" Back in Minneapolis, on Thursday nights we assemble bleach kits for addicts, and in late summer, we hand out condoms at the Minnesota State Fair. Memorial services mark the seasons; newsletters like *PWAlive* express feelings through imagery, poetry, and articles. These, too, were heady times, mostly somber, but not without a trace of dark humor, rebelliousness, and an uncanny closeness because of the common, shared experience.

Paul's Test Results

Paul, the night you finally told me, I left my apartment in a rush. Adrenaline pumped so hard throughout my body. Walking around Lake Calhoun three times that night, each time faster and more determined, the power of the adrenaline raced through my muscles. Tension built in my own body as I concentrated on yours; my heart pounded. Branches of trees, park benches, and ducks—I barely saw them—all viewed as obstacles blocking my way. I kept saying to myself, "I won't let this happen; I won't let him die," with teeth clenched, breath coming out in spurts, gulps, and snorts. As if I had any real power. As if someone would listen. How arrogant of me. Paul, you should have seen me. No, it's better that you didn't. I raged that night, the beauty of the park wasted around me. I didn't see it; I couldn't see it because all I saw was you with the number 1600, for T cells, plastered across your forehead. I tried to visualize that as you wanted me to—all those positive thoughts you required. I was also angry—very, very angry. I knew what was about to happen.

Conversation with Paul #5

"Paul?" I ask. We are sitting in his kitchen in our pajamas.

"Yes?"

"How is it that you can get up every morning?"

He starts to cry. "Now see what you made me do."

"I didn't make you do that . . . ," I say gently. "Aren't you taking antidepressants anymore?"

"No, I stopped."

Paul walks behind his kitchen counter and pulls out a slew of other meds. He shows them off to me, one bottle at a time. Then the AZT.

"So what is *that* like to take? Are there any side effects?"

"Yeah. Just one."

"What is it?" I ask.

Paul looks across the counter and directly at me. "This: EHHHHHHHHHHHHHHHH," he is screaming and does so until we're both bent over laughing, pj's soft against our skin, sleep still resting in the corners of our eyes. Still the same Paul.

Conversation with Paul #6

In his orange convertible with the top down, we drive out to lunch later that day.

"Paul?" I ask sitting beside him on the way to Sausalito.

"Yes?"

"I just want to talk to you about some things. But they're kind of hard to talk about."

"Go ahead."

"What about your drinking? Don't you want to stay as healthy as you can for as long as you can? Shouldn't you make a will?"

"It doesn't matter. None of it matters." He guides us between the traffic on the crowded bridge.

"It doesn't?"

"I'm dying."

After a few more miles, he says, "At my funeral, I'm going to make every single person there kiss me right on the lips."

We both laugh. I still worry.

After lunch, during which we fight over who is buying, we return home. Our car scurries across the Bay Bridge, wind forcing the hair back into our faces, tunes reverberating at top volume. The car, which he bought used, had special devices built into it, so that the gas pedal and brakes were hand controlled. The car, nearly airborne, must have looked from above like a metal speedboat, with the big blue on both sides of the pencil-thin bridge. This time both of us screamed as loud as we possibly could with abandon as we drove. No one could hear us. We knew this was one of the last times. That's why I had left one of the photo strips of Paul and me at the Woolworth's photo booth. We made three strips and I left one behind, so some person we would never meet would find them. That way, we would remain anonymous, immortal—forever fixed in a moment in time that only he and I would ever know.

60 Minutes

I spend most of the morning making lists, getting quotes on renting sound and camera gear on the phone as I attempt to calm my nerves. My work partner Kevin just informed me that we are crewing a *60 Minutes* program for CBS News in Cincinnati in two days. Although we've worked on network shoots before, this is a new show for us, so I'm fighting off excitement and nerves while pulling together details. The phone rings and I grab it, thinking it's probably a rental house calling me back or Kevin with more instructions.

"I've got some news for you about Paul," Molly, our mutual friend, says over the phone.

"Oh God. Is he back in the hospital again? Is it another round of pneumocystis?"

"No. Actually, Paul died. His funeral was in New York three weeks ago. I just found his address book and am calling people now."

Funeral! What is she saying? I just saw him this fall. He just called me a month ago on my birthday. He can't be dead. He is just supposed to get sick and recover, and get sick and recover—indefinitely—as he has been doing. He's not supposed to die in New York. I know what he did. He stayed alive through the winter so he could go back East and see his mom and sister—that's what he was up to. His message said he'd try to stop in Minneapolis on his way back home. Funeral in New York, three weeks ago, I can't even go to his funeral. It already happened. He *died!* How can he be dead?

After the call about Paul's death, I contemplated staying home and not doing this shoot. I hung up the phone and slowly walked to lunch. My steps were extremely heavy as I thought about what I should do. My face drained. My mind slowed to a sudden stop. I realized how pissed off Paul would be with me if I didn't take the job, so I went. He had recently given me a silver and turquoise bear pin. I wore it to the shoot.

I did the work in Ohio that next day, even enjoyed it—the long hours of lighting, setting up the cameras, coordinating with the other sound person. When Lesley Stahl arrived, the frantic pace began. I was perhaps quieter than usual—somewhat tucked within myself. The story was one of a series about environmental activists being targeted with violence. I talked with the woman whom we profiled. She was a young, undereducated single mother who raised concerns in her Cincinnati community about pollution from a chemical barrel factory situated next to a grade school.

I walked around her crummy apartment in the heat of that day, read the tiny encouraging notes she had written to herself on a bulletin board above her desk. She owned nothing really, but had led marches, had done public speaking, and more. Now bullets and bricks went through her windows, the family dog died after being poisoned, and she received hundreds of harassing phone calls. We interviewed her, walked by the barrel plant and filmed the angry workers there, and then moved on to a playground nearby. At lunchtime, I observed the neighborhood and noticed many out-of-work men, as a homeless lady walked near a cameraman, who slipped her some bills.

When the long day ended, I called Paul's sister from the airport because, coincidently, she lived in Ohio. We discussed the upcoming memorial for him in San Francisco.

The Apartment

I enter through the front door, like a million times before. This time I keep a watchful eye on it all—the woodwork in the lobby, the sound of the door closing, the feeling of stillness. I mount the stairs and absorb the feelings of melancholy. Once inside his door, I stand in the center of the hallway facing the living room. "Paul?" There is no answer, but he is still here.

My anxious hand barely reaches for the wall to steady myself. His smell still permeates the rooms, his furniture, the clothes in his closets, his books. He hasn't left yet. I simply stand there with fingers on the walls trying to make contact, calling his name for several minutes and then listening to the silence. Where is he? I try my hardest to conjure his image, to bring him back here, to get him to throw back his red hair and laugh. Command him to play a CD from his collection and dance alone, unencumbered in front of the fireplace. The music to blare out the windows with the steel gray curtains and onto Sanchez Street below, so that all the yuppies, ex-hippies, and newcomers can hear the concert of this once-vibrant young man.

I'm standing in his apartment. My fingertips moving on the walls, trace some kind of hieroglyphic narrative, trying to communicate. "Do you hear me? What are we supposed to do now? You weren't supposed to die. You were supposed to be the one who was spared. You were the smart one, the one with the degree in psychology. You taught me about living with a positive attitude, self-esteem, humor, responsibility, being honest. I heard you. I remember all of your different apartments, every couch and chair you ever had, the cats, your favorite foods, the practical jokes with your neighbors who now are my friends, the modern art that you adored, the goofy postcards you sent. I remember every anonymous fuck you had, since you were never able to center on one. All because you told me."

My message, among others, still on the answering machine. It contains a series of one-sided conversations from people trying to keep him from leaving. Each message becomes slightly more alarmed than the last, until people are hysterically calling out his name, as I am now, hoping that the strength of our voices would keep a ruthless god from taking one more person. Hoping God would say, "Enough. You can have this one. Your love is pure."

I'm frozen in Paul's apartment on Memorial Day. Kim and Jon come back and they, his final caregivers, graciously allow me ten minutes alone in his apartment. "Paul, are you here? Where did you go?" I touch the walls, breathe in his smell. Eventually, I become frightened by the silence, the finality, so I gladly let my friends back in. I'm here to pick out a few mementos before the flight back to Minneapolis and my new roommates at the big house on Dupont Avenue. There is to be a party tonight.

I look at various items. They are too big for the plane. No furniture—impractical, although I could have used the platform bed. Downhill skis? Not really. I collect a few books, socks, a vase, black-and-white towels, and a shirt. Then pack the cowboy pillowcases and hot pads I made him, a lamp, and one piece of art. This piece, one of a series of prints done in earth tones and white, created by a friend of his and John's, R. Anderson, whom I never met. Later, someone mails all the postcards and letters I've sent him from Minneapolis, which he saved.

Kim, Jon, and I make lunch from the remains of the food left over from the wake. Buckets of Hawaiian flowers surround us. We laugh while we eat. Submerge ourselves in him. We sit at his kitchen table; we use his plates and glasses. Make a toast and promise aloud to meet him on the other side. I run for the plane. When I arrive home in Minneapolis, I go directly to our living room. There, in our grand old three-story house, my five roommates and I prepare for a community party we planned long ago. The oriental rugs are rolled out of the way and crowds of people have already arrived, with more coming in. I change my clothes, put on makeup, come back downstairs, and dance for hours. Dance.

I Lie Here

I lie here in the bed next to yours. When my head turns, your body appears; I watch you sleep. My consciousness is beginning to fade. The flight was a long one, and I am in need of this nap. As doctors and nurses whirl by, we take our turns, me sleeping while you are in a much deeper state. We're letting go of all the sadness and turmoil that fills our minds. I glance over to watch you again; I wonder if you heard me come in. John, I've come to say good-bye.

Today is not a good day. While your mom explains to the psychiatrist and grief counselors how you and I moved her into that last apartment, tears find me. Sorry, John. I place both hands on my head, as if to admit surrender, and the tears become quietly unstoppable.

Your mom really relishes this story of us moving her, giving many details. The staff supports her and someone casually passes a Kleenex my way. Since I arrived a few days ago, my time with you has been rather cheery—visiting with our friends, hanging out with you. Now the seriousness of your illness has reached me. You know me so well. John, can you hear me? Do you know it's me?

Do you remember that night when I called you? After I yanked myself out of denial. It grew so strong that I have no clear recollection of how long I was not in contact with you. Then I called. You taught me about AIDS that night, not to fear it, but to know it. You told me a year ago that losing your independence was the hardest thing.

Then your voice got rather strange. Sentences became jumbled around and you would stop in the middle and repeat what you had just said, many times over. This really frightened me, John. Dementia. I didn't know it. I only knew I was losing you—sentence by sentence, word by word. I never thought your mind would be whole again, but it was. When I had last visited, you recovered it. How could that be? That the snarl of sentences clears into a straight path once again. Were you frightened? Did you realize the difference? When we spoke during the last visit, every word had a context, the order correct, the placement precise.

Six months ago we lunched at your mother's apartment, laughing, catching up on news while you tinkered with her music box. You gave me that photo of yourself in the green plaid shirt and cowboy hat. You were moving so fast in the photograph, there is a blur where you should've been still. You're still now.

———————

John, you gave me a birdcage once. It was made of wood, its white arches rounded at the top. So pretty. It was too nice for a real bird to mess up. I went to a florist and found a tiny decorative bird made of feathers. It occupied its new home happily. I still have it. The birdcage—I used to sit and study it. The shape, delicate design, its brightness, the way it looked so glorious in my San Francisco apartment in the late afternoon sun.

———————

Now I'm touching your sweaty brow, kissing your head. My fingers massage yours, John. I hear young men screaming and moaning in the distance, down the hall. They never reveal their faces, only voices.

I keep forgetting that you can't see me; you're blind now. Yeah, you look good. Just thin, very thin. Your breathing seems troubled. Let me call someone. They say your liver is going and the fluid filling your lungs, every half hour, needs to be sucked out. John, I swear to God, you still look handsome. Trust me, you look marvelous.

I've tried to prepare myself for a long time—when you had meningitis, then pneumocystis—but when the call came, it still stopped my breathing. I was surprised you were still alive when I got here.

John, I've got to get out of here. Out into the early afternoon sun, where I can get some air. When I try to stand, I slump back down. My legs don't work right. I'm still crying, and my legs seem elastic and wobbly. I can't seem to stand or walk, John. My body just won't hold me, and I suddenly feel so fragile and alone. Using my hands to hold on to the dull hospital walls, I limp slowly down a hall, oblivious to everything. Sorry, sweetie, I'll be back tomorrow.

You got pretty mad. The doctors and nurses keep telling us to be careful what we say. Hearing is the last of the senses to go, they warn. Hearing your brother talking across the room, you swung your twisted, broken body around sharply and shouted, "I'm not going to die!" You were so pissed. Your mind and spirit are so strong, but that body is just not available to you. I can't fix that. You can't live in it anymore. It becomes more useless by the hour, the minute. The rage is still inside you.

For a time, there is nothing. There is no way in and no way out. Just whiteness and light. Your eyelids fall. The room swirls around us. Head and body start to change color, and then, form. You fight back a little, John, but we know death is near. Resting necessitates this transformation. You've come so far and this is all you can do now. You're safe with us. We have you. Our faces receive each other, while the noise outside the room fades away. It's just us now. Like before. Now there is nothing.

Years March On

My experiences with AIDS, both in San Francisco and Minneapolis, grow heavy. I carry them with me until the weight simply prevents me from moving in any direction.

For every pair of black boots, I see dozens, hundreds more. Every blue jean jacket begets another, every cashmere sweater, every leather vest reflects the '70s. Every omelet, every mimosa, every green salad takes me back to similar aromas. Every convertible going over a bridge once carried me and a man like this one. Every musician, every psychologist, every antique dealer resembles those from before.

Every gay man who ever moves me from fourplex to cottage reminds me of one who moved me from Victorian to Victorian, duplex to duplex. Every man who listens to stories of my troubled romances, every man who comforts, every man who lets me lean on him feels like those I've leaned on before. Every giggle, every protest, every funeral, every walk on the tracks, every *Saturday Night Live*, every bird, every haircut, every flower reminds me of San Francisco—the city and the men.

Every art gallery, every airport, every donut shop, every drugstore, every beach filled with pairs of men reminds me of other pairs. For every Gregg, Ron, and Ms. Charlotte there was a John, Howard, and Mary. For every unemployment counselor, physician's assistant, and fundraiser there was an urban planner, a hospital administrator, and a waiter.

Every hit of pot, every glass of wine, every line of coke, and every microbrew brings back other times. Every camping trip, bluegrass festival, puppet show, or opera brings dozens of others into view. Every mustache, every beard, every bald head of a baker, a photographer, or a salesman brings me home to another time, place, and sequence of familiar faces.

For every writer, there was a writer. For every lover there was another lover. For every drag queen there were three drag queens. For every student there was a student. And for every dead gay man another one carries on. If only in my mind, if only in front of my eyes, if only in Minneapolis and St. Paul.

ACT UP SF

Kim and I stand at Castro and Market, two streets coming into crisp focus through the crosshairs of AIDS—ground zero, as it is often referenced. Tonight marks the first decade of AIDS in San Francisco. Kim and I unwittingly find ourselves stumbling into this demonstration while I'm visiting.

By now, in the mid-1990s, the disease has confronted us continuously since its start and wiped out our friends, neighbors, and coworkers as if they were annoying gnats on a summer evening, just brushed them aside with the wave of a strong hand. Our closest friends are all dead now, but AIDS keeps coming back. Despondency and fear rush to hit me squarely in my chest at this corner that has been the site of so many street fairs, concerts, Halloween parties, and times of frivolity. The corner once held crowds from the ornate Castro Theatre, buckets of fresh roses, the aroma of Italian food, and the sweetness of a bakery. There is no joy to be found here tonight.

The Twin Peaks bar, with its floor-to-ceiling windows, is now known as the "glass coffin" because so many of its gay patrons have died. Named for two great hills that afford the best view of the city, a sparkling chain of lights down Market Street, the bar stands at the tip of the intersection and gives a preview of all that is to come.

Tension heated up in the Castro District, as marchers were greeted by grossly excessive numbers of riot police. Some 200 cops were met by 300+ marchers.

Chalk outlines of bodies are being drawn in the middle of the street, much like the ones police mark at the scene of a crime. Hundreds of us surround them.

I feel my throat constricting, while Kim and I stand still, frozen in place, as the figures are drawn on the pavement before us, this corner as familiar to us as our backyards, as our dead friends' faces. A young person outlines the bodies of our friends, and their friends, and the friends of others in grotesque conceptual art. We feel the connection as if they are murdered right in front of us because we have lived so close, mere blocks from where we stand.

Some demonstrators attempt to "take" the intersection of Market and Castro, as the traditional symbolic show of strength in our own neighborhood. One group had intended to spray-paint a permanent quilt on the intersection.

Now the whistles begin to shriek. ACT UP members blow them continuously, spreading an atmosphere of urgency and alarm. I stare ahead solemnly watching, and yet my limbs shake and my head is in a state of confusion because of our chance meeting with this contingent in our old neighborhood.

Angry protestors sat down in the intersection, now in protest of the inordinate display of force by police on what is perceived as home turf. One by one, police arrested all those who sat in the street. The charge: inciting a riot and failing to disperse on command.

I find myself still trembling, still disturbed, unable to move. More than street theater or performance art, this scene is real and finally an outpouring of emotion from a community pent up with stifled grief. There had been no medical breakthroughs, no government plan, nothing to stop the onslaught. In this kind of repression ACT UP was born.

A 10-foot sidewalk, crowded with newspaper boxes and garbage, became a holding pen for 100 demonstrators and some unaware bystanders. Police shoved the crowd into this space and surrounded them on all sides. . . . Captain Cain (badge #1942), in an unprovoked act of violence, began swinging his nightstick. At least three people were injured, one who ended up in the hospital with stitches above his eye. . . .

Our neighborhood, precious because of the relationships we made there in our twenties, is under siege, and we feel powerless to stop it, much less understand all that has happened here tonight. On this spot, Cleve Jones, a political activist, had spoken before a memorial march of thousands to city hall after the assassinations of Mayor Moscone and Supervisor Harvey Milk. Now we stand at this same epicenter in the dark, still stiffened by the shock of death and dying that claimed those very people from the earlier times. A thousand men died in one year on just a few of these blocks. Cleve later created a quilt for them. We carried them, held them, washed them, fed them, and we're still mourning them.

The police began to "sweep" Castro Street. Many of those arrested were not involved in the demonstration.

I'm terrified by the anger, the outlines of death, the confrontations. Clutching each other, Kim and I both start to run, the sound of the whistles chasing after us. We run because of our own cowardice; we run to escape the police; we run for our own survival. This fight is ours as well, but we aren't always strong enough to stand up to it.

After the police left the Castro (some five and a half hours after the start of the march), the crowd that remained formed a circle and retook Eighteenth and Castro for twenty minutes of triumphant singing and shouting.

San Francisco Revisit, 2006

I return to San Francisco to connect with my past and face some things that have changed. Most of my old friends here have a two-night rule for sleeping over, since they get so many visitors. So I spend my trip hopping from one nest to another. It's what happens when you live in a city that is a tourist mecca.

Jim arrives at the airport to fetch me and we drive in style with his hybrid car. He says everyone in California has them. I met Jim's parents when I first moved to Minneapolis and through them, Jim and I became friends. He's forty-six years old and is all about meditation, Buddhism, and running. Some kind of computer whiz. Very assertive. He bought a duplex with a Canadian couple as a way to afford property in the Bay Area. Apparently, he didn't know about their screaming fights in the middle of the night before he signed the papers. So much for the sanctity of marriage.

We drive around the neighborhood and it feels quite surreal. It is late and yet all these little restaurants and cafés are open that I have never seen before, glowing with twinkling lights. I tell Jim how everything looks beautiful, to which he replies, "Everything looks beautiful in the dark . . . especially my car." Then he says, "Oh, we have to go down to ground zero," meaning Castro Street. I find his casual attitude a bit off-putting, but I have to remind myself that he's only lived here for ten years and probably doesn't know anyone who's died. Jim's nostalgic about places where he's lived in the Bay Area, and my memories are more than twice as old.

Later, I find a newspaper article on his kitchen table about how Castro Street is filled with glow-in-the-dark paper irises to commemorate the twenty-five-year anniversary of AIDS.

In Jim's neighborhood, at Dolores and Market, the streets are narrow and all the houses have grown together, as if one long facade. Streets tilt at 45-degree angles, like before. Gray, peach, and lemon boxes cluster close to cement walkways littered with an occasional shrub or an oversized jade plant. Narrow balconies beckon insiders to hang out, outsiders to peer in, or just act as an avenue for air exchange. I peek out the front window when I wake up and there are gay men everywhere! Jim tells me that there is a sex shop one block up, next to the women's bar Mecca, two marijuana buying clubs a few blocks down from there, and a needle exchange place. Not to mention that there is a huge pet supply store just a few feet away on Market Street.

I dash out of his duplex to head downtown this morning. Under my feet at the streetcar stop is a poem chiseled into granite, which goes something like this:

> *I am Cortez without a map*
> *and you are Leonardo da Vinci*
> *with your beard caught*
> *in the bicycle chain but*
> *moving forward anyway to*
> *the roar of your friends*
> *who say good luck!*

———

Elizabeth spends the night in a hospital with a dog bite gone bad, while I crash at her place. I recognize almost everything she has in her house, which she rents in noisy El Cerrito with the subway running directly above and behind her house. That famous blue oriental rug is here, wooden writing table, chipped plates. So now the three cats and I settle in. On the phone, she tells me, "I have a job, a house, and a car—I am luckier than ninety percent of the people in the world."

I can tell that there are many more women like me out here in Northern California—middle-aged, single, independent, educated. While I'm awed by the film and literary events in the Bay Area, I think about the crime and the price of housing both here in Oakland and in San Francisco and wonder if the heartbreaking compromises are worth it.

When I talk with EW, as I call Elizabeth, once more on the phone, she insists "I have time for my job, my siblings, and my friends, but that's all," brushing aside mention of relationships. Our discussion is frank, as she dissects her past dating of both men and women. I listen, appreciating her honesty.

Kim arrives and swoops me up, and we grab papaya salads, shrimp, and Thai barbecued chicken sandwiches as we head to her and Jon's house in Berkeley. The food here is so fresh and I feel totally indulged. We share the nitty-gritty of our lives and what's happened to us in the eight years since my last visit, things most acquaintances know nothing about. Within moments, Kim is sobbing in the car. I begin to remember how intense it is to visit here. We talk nonstop for hours, eating lunch behind their prairie-style home, passed down by a grandparent. We walk the neighborhood. Later, Kim lends me comfy flannel pj's. After I view the earthquake-proofing progress in their basement, which consists of reinforcement of the foundation, we settle in for a movie.

"Do you think I look like I've aged?"

"Yes."

"Last night you said I didn't."

"That was last night. This morning we're being honest," Tim says to me as I wake up Monday morning. We had spent the wee hours sitting in his studio comparing the process of creating a painting and composing a poem. At dinner the night before, Elizabeth, newly sprung from the hospital, and I hunkered down in one of the alcoves of Tim's new compound in Benicia. When we picked her up, she grabbed on to me. Hugging me strongly to her torso, she pulled me apart from her, looked at me closely, and then hugged me tightly again. Elizabeth has been caring for her sick brother in Portland, and the stress shows.

After dinner, we admire Tim's new paintings and I position my two friends toward each other. "He really likes to go to films," I tell her. "She loves going to movies," I tell him. She also instructs him on how to leave cat food outdoors without having ants devour it, a trick he appreciates as the owner of many a stray cat.

Tim struggles now with jealously from other artists, since his work gets more attention. Recently, he replaced his broken-down car with a new Camry from the sale of some paintings.

I spend my last day alone, going to the new de Young Museum to immerse myself in the quilts from Gee's Bend, wander through the African art wing, and see a vibrant Chicano exhibit on the lower level. I drag myself out at the last possible moment to re-create a photo of the Golden Gate benches that I took in the mid-1970s. Then I bus it to a streetcar, back to the Castro neighborhood. Running out of time. Crouching to the ground while waiting for transportation, I write in a notebook everything I see.

Racing now to visit three of the places where I, or friends, previously lived—the place on Church Street, and the one Casey and I lived at above the store, and last, 364 Sanchez. I duck in and talk with the manager of the Castro Theatre, a bookstore clerk, residents in several of the buildings where we had lived, all on my way back to the subway. It's great to see men holding each other in public again, hand in hand in the museum and on these streets.

At one of my old apartment buildings, I chat with a current tenant. "I lived here thirty years ago," I say. At the Sanchez apartment, which has since been gentrified, a man who lives there is less trustful of me. Palms and wild grasses are set into stone containers, while courtyards front turquoise-bricked walls near gates of black iron curved into half-moons. The trolleys and buses still define boundaries and borders, whether straight up the hills or bumpily straight along.

Later, I am filled with rage at the current tenants. "Don't they realize what happened in there?" My host, Kim's Jon, looks at me and says quietly, "Yes, I imagine they do." My gut tells me they are too young and too concerned about *now* to remember *then*. And that disturbs me.

The one person I don't see on this visit is my old roommate Casey. Our reacquainting phone call a few years later goes something like this:

"Hey, Casey! How the hell are you? We have a lot to catch up on. Glad you called," I say from the desk, the phone pressed against my ear. She had tracked me down on Google. "So what's happened to you after all these years? Did you and David stay together?"

"No, we are the best of friends, but we didn't stay together."

"I remember when you two got married. You eloped and took those pictures in someone else's wedding clothes after the fact and sent them to your folks out East. Where are you living now?"

"Oh, I had a great place down by the Duboce Triangle near the Castro that I lived in for seventeen years. It was a two-story Victorian that was rent controlled. I loved that place. A few years ago the building was sold and the new owner wanted my space."

"So what are you doing for work?"

"Actually, I just retired recently after working for over twenty years at the U—over in Berkeley." Then Casey paused. Somehow, I think she was trying to protect me from something. "I did financial work with AIDS."

"Wow. What was that like?"

"It was crazy. All the red tape from the university. I ended up paying for the HIV training and expenses, some in Africa, out of my own pocket. We had nurses and doctors submitting expenses all the time—it was nuts. I was wiring money left and right."

"I can so see you doing that. Why did you retire?"

"Well, there was a lot going on. I was going through all the trauma of having to move out of my house, so I just told everyone that the day after my birthday I was going to leave. They couldn't believe it, but that's what I did."

"Have you made peace with that?"

"Yeah. I had to get out of there. Everyone was dying around me."

Heal

_____

Here They Are

Here they are. John and Paul. This must be the kitchen. I can't really tell because the background is blown out, but from being there so often, I think they're in the kitchen. The color is weird in this one. I must have used a flash, or maybe I didn't take the picture. John is tending to a hanging plant, his arm reaching up and touching an ivy vine. He's looking up at it. His face is half in shadow, and I only see him from the chest up, one arm's cropped out. The shadow above his right eye creates a Groucho Marx bushy eyebrow. It's just an illusion. Paul stands next to John, but his arms are at his side. His young face, he must be twenty-five here, eyes calmly look straight ahead. He's got one long mustache and sideburns—needs a haircut. Yes, I think you can tell that his hair is red. Because of the color temperature, the entire image has an orange glow. My guys, doing their thing, together. John's actually wearing a ring here; it glows. I wonder who gave it to him. Neal? What year would this be, '78, '79? I guess John was always the doer, Paul the thinker. Apparently, I'm a doer and a thinker, as they were both my best friends. I think this is in the morning. I see sleepiness in Paul's eye. He did love to sleep.

John, Paul, don't worry—I haven't really changed that much. Still uncertain at times, constantly looking for community, although I've stopped sleeping around. Trust me, it's a good thing. You'd still recognize me, but my hair is much whiter now. I'm still up for a project though, like to do physical things. Still making movies, although this may be my last. Sometimes I'm a little melancholy, but mostly the same old me. I bought one of those new digital still cameras. Love it. By the way, we're still in Iraq, couldn't stop Bush from going to war. The Enron mess— corporate greed versus the "little people"—replayed . . . Guess what? I have a new place. It's an 1850s Victorian. Do you believe it? It's on the national and Minnesota historic registry. Huge. With bay windows, fireplaces, a butler's pantry. I feel at home here. And, hey. You'd love the old pie safe that I made into a bookcase.

ACT UP DC

On October 12, 1993, I fly to Washington, DC, to participate in a die-in. It's billed as a "massive AIDS wake-up call to Bush, Clinton, and Perot." I travel alone, but my uncle lets me stay at his place while he's out of town. At the Ellipse, an oval park south of the White House, most people chat with each other about where they traveled from to get here. While we're becoming acquainted, the chanting begins: "END THE AIDS CRISIS NOW." I photograph the march as linked arms three deep encircle the White House. I feel nurtured and safe within these arms. They may be strangers, but we share the same beliefs, the same passions. The signs and banners say it all—black background, pink triangle, white letters: SILENCE = DEATH. Some throw blood and human ashes onto the federal gates, the goal to hold these administrations accountable. I doubt that those in power will understand the significance of these very personal acts, but they are done all the same.

When the ACT UP whistles blow, thousands of us hit the ground, lying in a haphazard network of humanity. This time I don't run away, like Kim and I did from the Castro Street demonstration. The thought never crosses my mind. I hit the ground. Hard. There's a bit of nervous laughter from those on the ground beside me, then silence. As I lie there, motionless, more still than I've been in over a decade, among wave after wave of caring souls, I think about a generation lost. I think about the ones from San Francisco who lived in the Castro and walked the same streets I did.

I Would Have

Had I known they would all die, I would have stayed—made meals, easy ones since I wasn't a cook, surely tuna hot dish. I would have fought more with Paul about his vices, made Howie laugh by reminding him about the fancy art opening when my pants split open and I made him walk behind me all evening. I would have gotten to know Sue, Paul's sister in Ohio, long before the wake, and Howie's sister in New Jersey before she resented me for being able to receive a copy of his death certificate from the Public Health Department. I could have taken away some of the burden of care that fell to John's mom and brother, later to Kim and her spouse, Jon.

I would have liked to read to them. I'd read to Howie the newsletter put out by the hospital where he was an administrator. Or from a precious psychology book for Paul, who loved the intellectual stimulation of college. For John, from a trashy gay novel—he loved raunchy sex scenes depicted in words. I could have done it all.

Or could I? Negatives don't exist in this idealistic fantasy. No diarrhea, tumors, dying alone in a dark room, or despair. Neither do I deal with the anger or fear—theirs or mine.

I would have taken them for walks in the neighborhood, on sunny Castro or pulsating Twenty-Fourth Street, where Bud's (their favorite ice cream shop) was, or trips to Golden Gate Park to the Asian art museum, maybe the flower conservatory, a picnic to Stinson

Beach. But then again, there would have been times when they wouldn't want to leave home, their beds, get out of their pajamas. Long periods of time when they wouldn't want to see anyone, wouldn't answer the phone. Later, speaking only in gibberish.

We'd hear the roar of waves or cheering at an outdoor concert at the Berkeley Bowl, the silence and screams at Cecil's church, the pattern of their chatter after lattes. A sigh, that cough, the sound of a gentle kiss. In this vision, I see no squalor, no bloodstains, no loneliness.

I would have touched them often—putting my hand on the side of a lean face, a determined one. Body holding up body, mind holding up mind. Arms around the torso, fingers in their hair. Arm along their backs, eyes winking and holding theirs as tight as a top. A voice that drew their attention and comforted. I would have liked to do all of this daily.

But I couldn't. I wasn't there, except for a fraction of the time. I was naive, idealistic, and unprepared.

Forgive me.

Neal & Ben

We'd made a plan. The sanctuaries that had stood strong for over two hundred years would provide a meeting ground on the first Sunday after the next quake—the big one. Our plan came to pass, but certainly not in the way I had expected.

We depart early, before dawn. It's 2006. Neal, his partner, Ben, and I drive in darkness. San Xavier del Bac Mission appears like an alabaster mirage, shimmering in the distance just outside Tucson. While not the mission church I had anticipated returning to, San Francisco de Asís on Dolores and Sixteenth in San Francisco, this one shares its Spanish colonial origins and Franciscan leadership. Both were built in the late 1700s and survived centuries.

For many years I felt alone with the memories of what happened in San Francisco. But at some point I realized that Neal might still be alive. I tracked him down by sending a Thanksgiving card to his parents out East. That's how he came to call me.

Neal became my bridge between the living and the dead. Between my past and present, between San Francisco and St. Paul. Seeing him made me so joyful. At long last, someone I knew who could share the memory. Not another middle-aged white woman like me, but a gay man. We shared the experience of being in the

Bay Area at the same historic times of the mid-1970s. Neal had been there, known the same folks I had, loved them as I had. Both of us had moved before AIDS had really taken hold. We were lucky to survive, to remember, and to be able to reconnect.

For Neal, I filled in some of the details—John suffering from meningitis and later dementia, Paul collapsing on the tarmac. I even showed him a picture of Paul and me in Kim's living room in Berkeley, with the tumor protruding from Paul's neck, restructuring his face in an obscene manner. I wanted Neal to know every nuance, and he kept asking me questions and explaining things to Ben. My visit to Canada to see our old Hong Kong roommate Serena and toddler Cindy made for some light moments. I begged Neal to help me find them again.

Neal last saw his friends and old lover before their descent. Perhaps that was best. Neal had been doing precisely what he was supposed to be doing—moving in 1979 to Phoenix, meeting and loving Ben for twenty-five years. He was the one not surrounded by a city of dying friends; he was the one who found a partner and was allowed to love him. He was the one who was given a much fuller and normal life. Finding him gave me tremendous joy and hope.

I'm a single woman of fifty-six, so I watched the two men in awe at the kind of familiarity and ease that come from longtime companionship and love. Neal would make them each a bowl of oatmeal and have everything timed perfectly, so that the minute Ben walked into the kitchen after waking, it would be ready to eat— bowls steaming on the stove top, spoons poised.

They talked to each other throughout the day by cell phone right up until the moment they simultaneously walked through the door after work. It was funny because I spent time alone with each of them and both wanted desperately to know what the other had said about him. Neal wanted Ben to sweep the kitchen floor more often and Ben wanted Neal to be more spontaneous, they told me in whispers.

Ben showed me a photograph on his computer of a piece of land they owned in the desert, where they wanted to build their dream house. "Let me have Rosemary for a while," he said to Neal. Ben, with his yogic demeanor and shy manners, grew lively as he pointed out their future path along the dry earth, cactus, and mountainous skyline.

––––––––––

Now, in another part of the Arizona desert, we arrive at the mission. Scaffolding masks half of its exterior, but a few tourists and locals mix as always. We walk the grounds—up the hill next to the compound of buildings. Bells and booklets tell the history of this place, the *white dove of the desert*. A grotto reveals itself high above, no one up there but us, and a prayer fence. We wander for a while, above the monumental church and visitors. The grit and crude construction on this level hold part of the wildness of the landscape. Each of us slides deeper into our thoughts and silent talks with God. I stay within arm's length of Neal and Ben for the comfort.

Inside the church, we are transfixed by the beauty of the carvings, angels, and sacristy. One of the guys spots the hidden face of the devil in a Last Supper painting. "Oh, I see him now," I say, discerning that bold, half-invisible menace in the otherwise fraternal image. I doubt if everyone visiting the mission can see it, but I did.

"Do you want to cop a feel?" Ben whispers later while we kneel in pews. I didn't respond. Did I hear what I thought I heard? Then he repeats. I'm not sure what he means until he explains the significance of the old wooden St. Joseph statue. Prayers can be answered. The locals touch him, lift his head. He lies in an open casket along the side of the church. Ben and I approach, like the old man is a relative. We comfort Joe, touch his chest and shoulder. It has been awhile since I've been in a church, so my hand strokes Joe timidly. But, yes, I don't just want to look; I want to participate. So I touch his head. For Neal's good health, I whisper. (I never find out if his newly diagnosed leukemia is AIDS related. In fact, he is dead within a year.)

Neal buys a candle in the chapel gift shop, and we return to the large sanctuary to light it. I see other candles, angel faces, and hard, rough pews; I hear the voices of singing. Yes, we made it to the mission. The earthquake, our big one, is over and those of us who have survived make time for this reunion. I look over at Neal's profile. Other quakes rumble, but we have come at last to mourn our dead and give thanks.

We light our votive at San Xavier del Bac, this historic mission church, place the candle deep within the rows of dancing fires, and leave it burning.

Smoke Rises

"Kim, I think it's over here," I whisper.

"Think so?"

"Yes, this looks like the one." I'm staring at a house on a small tree-lined street.

We're standing close together, across the street from where I faced the perpetrator with the gun, twenty-five years earlier. We're a half block from Dolores Park in Eureka Valley. Young people are leaving their parked cars and returning to their apartments. It's a quiet street. I gaze at the space between the Victorians, in front of the garage, where the conflict occurred, where I might have lost my life.

"Right there, that's where it happened. Right next to those bushes. You see that lower flat with the Queen Anne windows? That's the apartment. Stephen came out of that place to rescue me."

I think of his kindness, and I wonder what became of the other man—the man wearing a yarmulke and carrying a sawed-off shotgun in his carpetbag. Whatever I did that night, and I tried many different ways to change the outcome, I learned that I would do whatever is necessary to preserve my own life.

"Here, take one of these," Kim says. She has pulled a few Chinese prayer papers from her pocket. We hold them and light each on fire while standing quietly at the scene of the crime. The smoke rises from the thin, colorful papers and with it our sadness for the loss of innocence that night long ago. I also pray for any women he may have assaulted afterward, since the police were never able to apprehend and arraign him for his crimes.

Body Work

In the silence of a room, my back traces the boundaries of the massage table. The practitioner's hands rise above and push my flesh from side to side. My neighbor and friend is going to die today of AIDS. My limbs are kneaded—arms first, then legs. No words here. I feel my torso begin to shake. The room becomes invisible—all that white. While he pummels my back and neck, I begin to sob.

MAP

A small group, including me, then a thirty-year-old woman formerly from San Francisco, puts on the first Minnesota AIDS Walk. Our day begins with a 5 a.m. breakfast, then on to deliver porta potties, helium tanks, tables, and supplies to each refreshment station along the route. Two bridges across the Mississippi River are decorated, along with Minnehaha Park, where the walk begins. Volunteers collect pledge money and introduce The Firm, a fitness center, which gets the crowd stretched and ready to go. When it's all over, we same tired volunteers clean the park and pack away the tanks, tables, chairs, and balloons until next year. Dick, a sixty-year-old mailman from South Minneapolis, puts on a sundress and his red pumps and we all go party afterward. Each year when Dick puts on those pumps, we know the Walk is over.

A friend, Susan, and I organize the Thursday Nighters, a group of Twin Cities volunteers who meet each week in the brown room with the stained ceiling on Franklin Avenue to send out mailings, pack bleach kits for addicts, put condom packs together for State Fair goers—whatever the staff asks of us. Twenty-five years later, the group with a revolving regiment of volunteers, still meets.

One night, we were given a few boxes of a man's final belongings to divide among ourselves. There were Christmas ornaments, odd things. I took a little rubber alligator and put it in my bathroom. That way, when I see it, I can think about where it came from and the connections I've made with other Thursday Nighters. In a way, one man's life continues.

The annual holiday party at MAP, which began with just a handful of people, becomes a solemn occasion when we note who is missing. The singing of "Silent Night" brings tears to everyone's eyes, while people hang on to each other as a sign of solidarity in a circle warmly formed. I realize that the only times I attend church are for memorials and the annual interfaith service for those still living with AIDS.

I produce a video for MAP called "Safe Sex, Lies and Videotape," in which I record every cheap gag I can think of to get folks to laugh. I include uneven, wild camera zooms into a staffer's hair, a stand-up routine in a convenience store/gas station next door to MAP with the AIDSLine counselor/narrator holding a dildo as a mic. It goes on from there, to a whipped cream sequence with Eric, MAP's founder, a close-up look at what is in the center's refrigerator, and fake scenes of a police raid. I stay up all night editing it with the volunteer coordinator. "Safe Sex" brings howls at the annual party and is later shown to all new volunteers.

Circle

I joined a support group and cried whenever I said your name, Paul. I know you don't like hearing this. Yet you need to know. We've always been honest with each other. I sat with that group for three years, the one in the small room at Abbott Hospital. You could have facilitated that group, with your psych background. Mothers would be frantic—afraid of AZT. Whole families would sometimes show up in our room while at the hospital during an emergency, never to return. Mostly, we were sisters. Sisters, losing their brothers. I, the only one grieving a friend. But you were my brother, Paul.

So many facilitators—they kept dying or leaving the country or having babies or enduring surgeries. We wept for them too. You should have been there; it really helped me. Were you there? Did you come with me? Could you travel like that, through parking ramps, across deep pockets of snow, past the hospital McDonald's, and into that very small room? The one down the hall from the chapel that no one ever went into. The one not quite big enough to hold all of the emotion. Were you there with us? I wish you could have told me, if you were.

Days of the Dead

These are my dead: Paul, John, and Howard. I cling to memories of these closest friends dancing, laughing, and sitting on green sofas with their cats, long white candles on a bed stand, a ten-speed bike propped up against a bedroom wall. I watch as red sores begin to cover their heads; tumors protrude from their necks; blindness takes over. Their thinness gives way to the internal collapse their bodies endure. What once was meticulously groomed is ravaged.

Paul insists that I visualize the number 1600 across his forehead: an amount of healthy T-cells he wants, to make it through another month (800 is normal; anything under 300 is suspect). I try hard to make this elusive number transfer from my thoughts to his body. I soon learn a person can live for many months with a T-cell count of zero. This amazes and pleases me.

Paul collapses in an airplane idling on the runway heading back to San Francisco after a visit with his mom and sister out East. An ambulance takes him to a hospital, where he dies within hours. The funeral is in Buffalo, New York, his hometown. His mother tells her family and friends that her son died of cancer.

I send John a large plastic bunny rabbit that I find at a hardware store, a book called *The Wisdom of Insecurity*, and an afghan. We visit and he seems shell-shocked. His bout of dementia causes his words and sentences to collide and scramble in ways I can't rearrange into a cogent pattern. Strangely, his sanity returns but his doctor dies.

He says this matter-of-factly because each day now more people are dying, so much so that it is difficult to feel anything anymore. With no time to process, we accept and move on. Regrettably, I do this with his death as well, returning to grieve many years later.

I've lost track of Howard, the hospital administrator who once was a physical therapist and my good friend. He always wanted me to photograph him nude. I was too shy, however. Now I hear he's on the lecture circuit. Next someone tells me he last saw him in a hospital bed, but he doesn't remember which facility.

In order to find out if Howard is still alive, the public records office instructs me over the phone to put in writing his full name, state of birth, and approximately what year he may have died. I tell them he was my friend.

The Public Health Department confirms my fears when an envelope arrives that includes his death certificate. A fault line within me splits apart as I read the details revealed in the document within my quaking hands.

I examine the photographs I took—his angel face, curly dark hair, and serious eyes. I send these prints to his sister in Philly. The address is on the document—next of kin. We talk on the phone once. While I'm sick with the flu in bed watching the NCAA basketball tournament, she calls and later describes his memorial at the San Francisco Jewish Community Center. Howard's sister tells me that they read my letter aloud at their Passover Seder. Later, Howard's relatives accuse me of misrepresenting myself as a family member to obtain the death certificate and are bitter despite my denial, cutting off all contact.

On my refrigerator, I keep a photo of Howard, the one where he stands, beautiful as he was, with his books.

Quilt

The Names Project AIDS Quilt, with its miles of fabric stretched as wide as a city itself, inspires me to use color, drama, and mood to represent the different people I've known who have died of this disease. The designing and sewing of panels is a private act followed by public viewing.

Patterns of swirls and spirals end abruptly to express new designs in opposite shades of black, white, and gray. Imperfections in the printing of my fabric only add to its depth. I've kept this yardage for thirteen years, using it alternately as a curtain or tablecloth. Its sheerness makes it almost transparent. I fashion Paul's name out of white cotton.

I leave John's 1950s floral drapery fabric—green, burgundy, and gold—on my floor for weeks, not wanting it out of my sight. Eventually, it flies away and lands in classrooms, churches, and stadiums with the others, a multitude of others.

Turquoise and sand make up Howard's quilt design. I find serenity in the silkiness of the rayon, and the colors recall desert, mountains, and cactus.

These are the three of whom I dream. I encode secret messages into the six-by-three-foot quilt panels, with a tiny portrait on each. Then, to help me let them go, I make miniature versions in inches instead of feet, using the same fabrics and teensy letters so that I have a replica of them to keep, wrapped and secured, in a silver tin my mother gave me.

I work on one panel for a stranger too because that's how AIDS has changed me. It reminds me of the importance of community. We can take care of each other.

When George became ill, he returned to the small town on a lake in northern Minnesota, where he once lived. As he lay dying, wolves gathered nearby and howled each night. After he died, they grew silent and left. I respond to a request for volunteers, and so a group of us, all strangers to each other, make a piece of art to honor George's life. Our panel includes mostly waves of blues and greens, a scattering of paw prints, and the words of George's story written along the edges.

Soon all of these panels, including the four I worked on, find their way to the Ellipse, an oval park south of the White House, as the AIDS Quilt travels from city to city, town to town. Making the journey to DC several times, I walk among the panels and marvel at the variety, the vitality, and the virtue of the images that spread out for as long and as wide as I can see. Some are garish and whimsical. They have teddy bears attached. Some are exquisitely fashioned by expert stitchers, and others project casualness, like the T-shirts that adorn them. I swoon and stumble among a blizzard of intimate personage. Each step and each name calls me closer to the ones I know, the ones I lost.

World AIDS Day

Winter renders another bitter lesson to its Midwest citizens. The snow is deep, the air brittle. On December 1, 1989, World AIDS Day, a handful of artists gather along the banks of the Mississippi River for a predawn service. I join them in this frigid observance. We want to throw names of those we are remembering into a roaring bonfire, but the below-zero temperatures hinder us, so we speak our friends' and family members' names amid the tree shadows to the winds, the hot sparks and the frigid exhaling of our breath swirling around us.

Then we hike along the trail, hills, and ravines dotted with votives until we hear nothing but the cracking of the ice on the water below the bridges we come upon. A burning pallet is set afloat in the open river a distance away. White surrounds our bodies. It's daybreak. Bitter coldness, along with a newspaper reporter, joins the dozen or so of us. I don't know anyone, but that never stops me. I welcome the chance to be among strangers. Every town is a new town for me, every stranger a potential friend. Here, we are marking this day together, while the masses sleep or prepare for work. AIDS and its thievery motivate us to leave our warm beds. Never an early riser, I savor the beauty of the snow and candles, the power of the names and fire, the simplicity of the floating pyre. The brief rituals begin and end quickly, but solemnly. All of this occurs among St. Anthony

Falls, the resident donkey of Nicollet Island, and the commerce of the Minneapolis Farmers Market.

This is my home now.

I Am Released

I'm losing consciousness, lying here on a small table wrapped in thin gauze blankets, eyes closed, listening to slow music. A young woman places a hot towel on my face as she rests her hands nearby.

A fabric curtain of warm moisture drops over me. All is forgiven. For a time, not even thought exists—only a feeling of comfort and relaxation. All is forgotten.

Oil runs down my arms and her hands feel confident as they rub the warm elixir over my body. A corner of a chandelier is revealed when I open my eye slightly. Where am I? She whispers something, but her voice fades and I miss her words.

Through the steam and intimacy of the room, softness finds me. Each venture leads to further un-layering, less posturing, and more letting go. I wonder what she thinks of me. Quiet prevails.

A cool liquid reaches cheeks, chin, and forehead. I rest peacefully, unencumbered. Healing oils penetrate my skin as I hear her gently encourage me to breathe deeper. Head slightly raised, my shoulders kneaded into submission. Calmness spreads like honey. The mind settles now. My limbs fluid, body rested and yet aware. An aura of golden light appears amid the whiteness. Who am I?

The warmth of the towel, the touch of a hand, a cover on my eyelids—each resonates a feeling of care. A young woman attends to the needs of someone twice her age. I now play the role of the older woman, but only on the outside of my body. The markers—

the age spots, the wrinkles, the swollen and red hands—belie the still-youthful interior landscape I inhabit.

The white muslin room opens itself and I am released.

Sunflowers

My sunflower garden hangs here in my bedroom. Merely four glassed-in sunflower images stalk that sliver of a wall. Robust, glorious, fading, and then withered—I watch each stage again and again. When standing close, I see the cycle repeat—camaraderie, revelry, wonder, surrender. Each stage a gift.

Execution of Justice

"COP: We been workin' this job three generations—my father was a cop—and then they put—Moscone, Jesus, the mayor—Jesus—Moscone put this N-negro-loving, faggot-loving chief telling us what to do—he doesn't even come from the neighborhood."

Execution of Justice, a play about the murders of San Francisco Mayor George Moscone and Supervisor Harvey Milk opens fall 1986 at the Guthrie Theater in Minneapolis. I take my place in the audience and marvel at how the director and playwright, Emily Mann, brings all the elements together. She includes dialogue from the actual trial transcripts and a cast who represent all the principal players in the tragedy. Sister Boom Boom, a black lesbian activist, a mom, and a beat cop were added to the mix. During the performance, several large screens descend and we watch actual footage from the memorial march. To see its enormity, solemnity, from another context—from outside of it and perceived as art—proves amazing. At the time, we were so vulnerable. We took our leaders for granted. Then we stood in the cold real streets of our own city and realized what we had lost.

Diane Arbus

Phil gave me a cast-iron frying pan that I use to this day. He tied a brown velvet ribbon on the handle that I saved for years. On one of my birthdays, he gave me a book by the photographer Diane Arbus, inscribing it with the sentiment, "In the hope that someday not too far away, your snapshots will get this good and then maybe you'll quit all that fucking horseshit about your womanhood. The photographs speak for themselves."

My reacquaintance with her work takes place on a free Thursday night viewing at the Walker Art Center in Minneapolis. Although many of the photographs have been committed to my memory, several of them I've never seen. Seeing the images with a running narrative that reveals much of Arbus's personal life gives the work much context; and at my midlife stage, I can see more that is unsettling and disturbed in her life than that of her subjects.

One image strikes me in particular. It is a black-and-white shot of a young girl selling plastic orchids on the streets of New York City at night. The innocence and beauty of this child and the mystery of her circumstances pulls me in. Like her, I face the dark and an unknown threat. She looks directly into the lens, as do I, and as do many of us. I want to know what became of this girl. I want to know whatever dangers she encountered during those long nights, she survived. I want to know she is safe now. I tell myself she is.

Films

Being able to see my friends again in these films as they were in their twenties, especially when they didn't survive their thirties, is gratifying but also heartbreaking. I thought I'd know these people for the rest of my life. To lose them so early was incomprehensible to a young woman who believed we were all immortal. Soon I became immune to the pain, as I could not process the reality of AIDS fast enough. We just kept moving forward, staying in the present. I talked to friends on the phone, visited them when possible, sent gifts.

The films I made give me a pristine portrait of friends in their healthy and carefree days. That's how I choose to remember them.

John Waters

John Waters peers over the young crowd gathered at the University of Minnesota's student union. Standing room only. Wiry, he talks fast, telling us he's had to give up most of his vices now that he's a middle-aged man. Funny. Still very funny. He talks of the late Divine and his own first mainstream film, *Hairspray,* and of working with Patty Hearst. How Winona Ryder and Johnny Depp were too young to get married, so they called it off. Baltimore, his hometown, is where most of his creativity hatched and he recalls how his career grew. His latest film, *Polyester*, has gone mainstream too. Well, not exactly. Funny, I feel like he and I are the oldest ones here. Funny, we are.

Headline

On August 13, 1998, the *Bay Area Reporter* runs a front-page headline "NO OBITS." The *Reporter* made a practice of publishing both obits and photos. It is the first week since the epidemic began in San Francisco during the early 1980s that no AIDS deaths were reported to the paper.

Tanners Lake, Minnesota, 2006

I've been living on this lake for a year now. It's a small lake just ten miles north of St. Paul, here in the Midwest. Tanners Lake. No one can tell me where its name comes from, but here's what I do know: The center is about eighty feet deep, lily pads sit in a circle in front of my cottage, while ducks and birds of all varieties congregate. A group of houses, both large and modest, ring its shores and the lake's waves continuously move until stilled by winter.

Simply, I wanted a quiet place to be for a while. One of the few remaining original 1950s cottages in Oakdale, this home affords me 450 square feet in which to ruminate and write. But its red brick hearth cannot warm me enough, nor can its moss-green walls contain all of the feelings and thoughts of another time in my life.

Tanners, a quiet lake with fishermen, swimmers, and a continuously changing companion to canoe its surface, settles my spirit like no other place ever has and for that I'm grateful. Shifting waves create a rhythm for my existence, as the heron perched at the end of my worn dock begins a morning with an explanation point, and the alternating quietness and bird calls soothe my otherwise harried brain of daily worries—a job I'm not quite happy with, a man I can't figure out, a schedule out of control.

Today will be unseasonably warm, 65 degrees, for a day this

claustrophobically close to November. Last chance for me to be outdoors, touch up the paint on the back porch, rake some leaves, tidy up the garage. Autumn affords time to prepare for winter, as summer gave the time to celebrate a year gone by.

These seasonal transitions remind me of several years I spent in San Francisco, especially the autumns and chills of winter—in the 1980s AIDS brought winters without parallel. Each took a turn.

As the sky lightens up, I can see the lake more clearly. Mist moves quicker now, like tiny clouds across a fluid sky. The icy sections are more clear, presenting themselves like fragile islands. If we do reach the mid-40s this weekend, they'll undoubtedly disappear temporarily until back for good. What foliage is left on the trees shows itself on the other side of the bay. The weeping willows are mostly golden, while my own trees at home on this side of the lake have turned into skeletons reaching desperately across the yard. Mornings are the best viewing of the lake. Often I'm late for work due to my prolonged pauses at the door, like today, when I linger in purple-and-white embroidered pajamas.

The spray hovers over the lake this morning. Ripples of water move stubbornly, slowly. Just a smattering of leaves, while the remaining circles of foliage await my bagging. A lantern hangs on an iron staff at the point of my land.

It's almost dark now. Bare branches crisscross the grayish-blue hood over Tanners Lake. Shadows of treetops across the bay mingle with the waist-high brush and the remaining grasses, soon to lose their shades of green. I see lights illuminating windows on the other side and atop houses too far away to identify. My lantern shines too. I had to jostle it a bit to get it going. But it is burning brightly now. Reflections of the light scoot across the blackness, reflecting phantom fires and imagined full moons; in fact, the sky, darkening by the moment, lies burdened with heavy clouds. Like that dark sky, I carry my losses and their weight.

The sun flatlines across Tanners Lake. Once the burgundy and gold drapes are pushed back, splotches of light lie across the textured sofa. There's very little wind this morning, but the frigid air awaits. Animal footprints prance across my yard, then longer and deeper tracks cut across the lake beyond. No decipherable boundaries now, all is white. One large mound of snow settles where the firewood lies buried, as if all inside are in deep sleep.

With our first snow of the season on the ground, yesterday I reluctantly inched toward winter myself. First the corduroy pants. Next the sleeveless shirt (the hot flashes are running about every twenty minutes now), followed by a zipped-up sweater, then the black wool jacket, and topped with a soft tam and scarf wrapped several times around both neck and torso. Oh, and the duck boots. The new gloves are not nearly warm enough.

It's the wind that makes it feel like only a single digit above zero.

The birds come early—alone, in pairs, or groups of four or six. Intermittently flapping their wings in place, they hover just above the water's edge. Surprisingly, they take their time, although the water must be frigid now. The birds remain each day until the last minute before the lake freezes. They hang on as long as possible, probably reluctant to leave their home and denying that this time of change has come.

All the yards say the same thing: summer was here once. Pontoons are anchored cockeyed, hastily covered with tarps. Wooden swings, wishing wells, and whirligigs sit stiff and cold. Docks haphazardly rest near gazebos and screen houses, which look strangely out of place in the snow. There's an old Hudson gasoline pump at the end of a driveway.

It's that odd time of winter now. The novelty has worn off. The snow isn't fresh or attractive. I feel claustrophobic and want to just jump on a plane and get out of town. Every house and neighborhood looks drab, colorless. It's hard to beat the hopelessness out of all the gray days. They stumble over each other and we through them. The days are humorless, repetitive, and without distinction.

I know I can't stay here, just as I know I can't grieve my dead friends for the rest of my life. My time here is finite. It matters—the grieving matters. It serves a purpose and it will end.

Everything is still at the moment. In back, the icicles hang like knives until I break them off, just because I can, and reverse their direction turning them into swords. I suddenly feel more powerful. Gloves or no gloves, I find the car, spend thirty minutes scraping windows, moving drifts with my forearms, listening to the uneven gurgles of the fan when I turn on the heater, and finally set the engine in motion. Careful not to back up too far, I attempt the steep hill, dodging snow, ice, and gravel, and after several attempts back and forth, changing gears, riding that car like a wild stallion, I successfully gun it up the hill and head off to work.

Even on the coldest morning the melting has begun.

Stubborn they are—these flakes. Fragile, alone, yet together they form a mass with a strong agenda, a voice of beauty, a symphony of soundless adventure. This to be my last winter here. I am a snowflake too. Dancing, dizzy with wonder, confusion, and happiness. Let me fall. Let me live. Let me rest.

It's evening now. A haze drifts over the landscape—snow-laden yards, icy lake, stark tree branches. Over the weekend I watched a small bulldozer smash and tear up the ice in front of my cottage. "I'm having my shore done," said my neighbor Corrine on the phone. A crowd of boulders sat hidden behind her car at the end of the public access road, which hugs the fence on my right side.

When I squint harder, I see the workmen abandoned the idea of bringing the boulders through the ice break. Instead, indentations in the snow indicate where the rocks were dragged, like limp and heavy bodies, across my property. At the lake's edge, the wide gash festers, like the wound it is. It's there. You cannot see this place without knowing it, seeing it. Stretching across the entire frontage, it is so prominent, so invasive, so deep.

Amid the white, hazy landscape, this abrasion marks me. Its dark interior and jostled, sharp edges remind me that I cannot look away, nor can I deny the suddenness and fury of fate. As disturbing as this is, I know that out there in the cold the thinnest fiber forms a layer with which to mend the gash and that over these days and weeks it will be contained, forming a new fabric within itself, eventually to rejoin the lake as a whole.

The diagonal trail from which the boulders were rolled will eventually be covered with enough new snow to make this previous journey invisible. But I'll know it was there. In my mind I can sense each boulder—large, small, or obtuse—making its way in front of me and over me and through my yard. Yes, no matter how faint the trail gets, I will know they were there.

New Year's Day

It's a crisp day at the cottage. I sleep until 2:30 in the afternoon, which is a complete aberration for me. The night before was spent watching fireworks set off in a friend's driveway, a movie, and a quick peek at Dick Clark in New York, his speech slowed by a stroke but his stubbornness still presenting hopeful quips to signal 2006.

Now it's nearly 3:30 and I dress quietly, pulling on a black wool jacket and handmade scarf, stepping out into the snowy yard sans gloves since it is balmy at 30-something degrees. Forty-five minutes later, I'm pulling up to a condominium complex in the center of the city. In my hand, I'm clutching a flyer that reads "Sacred Circle Dance, Newcomers Welcome."

I open the iron gate, walk the brick steps to a door, and follow signage up a set of stairs. People turn toward me, smiling. We're standing in a large empty room with a vaulted ceiling and wooden floor, two windows on the far side, four banks of lights on the ceiling. In a corner, near the stairs, a couple of chairs and a small couch are covered with coats. I take mine off and look around. People introduce themselves. "Have you done any kind of dancing before?" "How long have you been coming here?" And so on.

At 4:30, the group moves to the center of the space, forms a circle, and holds hands. A man named White Ash laughs, bouncing the two strands of colored beads around his neck, and he introduces the first dance. He shows us the steps and we practice them several times. Then he starts the music and we begin. It is a Greek dance. As we start, I look around the circle. When not checking out the footwork of people opposite me, I glance into the faces spinning past.

Faster and faster we spin. Layers of clothing fly off until we drip with sweat and breathe hard between songs, and I cannot believe my own thirst. Some dances are more difficult. My steps falter a bit, but no one minds and the rhythms change with each song. New music joins old dances and old songs lift new dances. From our simple beginning dance, begun after a short meditation, to complex step work aligned with music that beats faster as we go, the circle and its participants begin to blur. Hands become moist, holding on to other hands. Sweaters and sweatshirts lie scattered on the couch, steps, and chairs until dancers remain glistening in the barest of dresses, sleeveless tees, and dainty tops.

Step together step, step together step. My feet move first right then left. Rhythms and music blend and change with each dance—Latvian folk songs, fifteenth-century troubadour, American bluegrass. We holler, bringing our hands above where their shadows play around a skylight, our hips gyrating and undulating as we move back out to re-form and move again to the right. The hand in mine is moist but my hot flashes are nicely timed to match the sweaty dance's end.

My weight shifts from right to left. I am to feel like a tree, swaying slightly in a circular motion until the next section of the dance begins. In those moments, we become lone trees clustered against the wind, but rustling slightly, private thoughts blowing through our brains, limbs at our sides, but still joined by the branches.

We are one. We are many. We are together. We are alone. We move. We feel. We contemplate. We are silent. We stand. Stand tall, erect, and we hold back the wind with our trunks. Hold it in our limbs. Nuzzle it with our faces. Feet planted solidly on the wooden floor, we sway. Step together step. Sway, sway, sway, sway. Step together step. We rise.

At the potluck downstairs, I chat with more new people. Two men standing behind the kitchen island kiss, one with his arms firmly wrapping the other's waist. Rachel and her husband set out their cheese, salami ground with wild rice, and Ghirardelli chocolate miniatures. I sit on a couch with two women and chat. They confess this is their first time as well.

I rush out to my car to see if I have a lighter shirt, and when I pass the windows to the townhouse on my way back, I see the group from the outside. Twenty souls, standing and lounging on Andrew's mission furniture, all engaged in animated conversation. What I didn't notice while I was inside is a giant rainbow flag hanging from the ceiling above the kitchen island. With spotlights shining through it, even though the fabric is sheer, the colors are bright and I see the kind of community that I want to live in. Straight and gay, men and women, couples and singles in one large space together.

When we hear voices upstairs singing, we head back up. Only candles light the space. The dancing we do by touch and memory. As we step in and rock on our heels, the arms go up and soon rest on the shoulders of those adjoining us. This feels natural. Shoulder to shoulder, we slowly rotate.

About a dozen of us remain. We sway. We do an ivy step; we hold onto each other's pinkie fingers while dancing with candles. The silence creates a deeper normal. The steps and notes hold, hold us in place and slow our thoughts. The music saturates our psyches and we focus on our movements, ancient ones that lead us to connect with other souls in other places and with each other now.

Here We Are Again

Click, click. Breathe.

The pose is broken; I am closer now and everyone, almost, is laughing. Casey in full laugh. Kim has moved closer, one hand on hip and the other covering her mouth. Paul is kneeling on the chair, both hands on the seat, his eyes twinkling and his face in giggles. Neal behind him is in motion—clapping, leaning to the left behind Paul. John, my precious John, is a blur, arms at his sides, jacket off, his face still serious, out of focus. I took the pictures. I was there.

Epilogue

Prayer

My own return to prayer began in the early to mid-1980s when I saw the bodies of my close San Francisco friends disappear like fish piling up in a wharf-side basket. In the final hours, bright eyes shining, staring up at me as if to ask the inevitable "Why?" Consequently, the '80s proved to be the most difficult decade of my life.

Before the public even knew about AIDS, the virus had infected all those young lovers in my adopted town. They themselves and the rest of us had to invent new ways of grieving and honoring their spirits, of mostly men in their twenties and thirties, men who were just out of college, being abandoned in scores by their parents and turning to their friends to help them die. It was in coming together, whether it be at the unending memorial services, delivering holiday stockings to people with AIDS, or doing fundraisers by biking through the streets, that we found hope. Our strength lay in conneccting with each other and forging new allies. It was the shared recognition of our vulnerability, our humanity, that helped us face so much death.

As a child, I had marched in a solemn militia out of Sacred Heart of Jesus Catholic Church on a spring Milwaukee morning, chapel veils fluttering with just the precise amount of movement. Each girl shimmered in her blue uniform skirt, virginal white socks and tops, shiny saddle shoes. Moving like miniature Madonnas, hands held in prayer, singular girls transformed into meadows of petite bluebells, ones with sweet songs on their breath and the omnipresent lace crowns upon their countenance.

The progressive Franciscan nuns at my high school, St. Mary's Academy—which began as a women's boarding school in the 1800s and was declared a nuclear-free zone in the late '60s—shaped me as well. Music, art, and community helped me grow. We held our own be-ins, drank grape juice while dressed in homemade togas at our Latin class feasts, and rode in tricycle races as our big brothers and cousins went off to Vietnam. I sang "We Shall Overcome" and "Kumbaya" for the first time. And each May the entire student body—a blanket of plaid skirts, boxy brown jackets, crisp white blouses, and penny loafers—surrounded a Maypole, where seniors gleamed in long white formals and one special girl dressed in wedding attire rose to the top of a staircase to honor Mary and become the bride of Christ.

So which prayer paths did I use as an adult? Whatever I was able to get my hands on. I prayed while sprinting repeatedly around Lake Calhoun in a complete rage. I prayed while lighting a menorah in a support group for family and friends of people with AIDS. I prayed for God to help me stand up and walk when my legs failed me as I attempted to leave a hospital in which my dear friend John lay blind and in a coma, with bile choking him and morphine killing him. Unbeknownst to me, Howie lay just doors down, exhaling his last breaths.

I prayed with a candle in my hand on windy nights every Memorial Day, as bells tolled in Loring Park in Minneapolis and in Golden Gate Park in front of the windmills to a small gathering, where I told stories about Paul, my soul mate. It took three years of daily devotion for me to realize I was powerless to keep him alive. I prayed while writing a grant, which brought me out to see him for the last time, while I watched a film festival across town and drove through the decimated Oakland hills, days after a mammoth fire left hundreds homeless and consumed every structure in its path.

I prayed to be snapped out of denial. I prayed out loud, when I heard of another man's death on the radio, slamming my fists on the dashboard while I argued with God about why Jack was taken. I prayed as thousands marched in flickering brightness to the reflecting pool of the Lincoln Memorial, including my Uncle Bob, who had remained closeted during his government military career and that night was marching for the first time. I prayed while laying fruit, photos, and marigolds on a Day of the Dead altar built on my kitchen table. Also at the National Cathedral, where gay men and others with AIDS accepted the laying on of hands.

I prayed for direction in knowing what I could offer the people I knew. My resources were limited, but I wanted to help. I found myself praying that my own HIV test would be negative, since I had slept with bisexual men. I prayed each time I revisited my old neighborhood. With each step and glance into a familiar window, or storefront, or stranger's face. Thoughts of the thousand men who died within a six-block area in one year, and the hundreds of skeletal figures who went on living, proved to be beyond my ability to process or accept. I prayed when Howard's death certificate arrived one day in my mail, and when a neighbor we finally located in a nursing home spoke gibberish because of dementia, and while awaiting HIV results of an AIDS Ride staff member, whom I had just met.

Unfolding the quilt at the Metrodome for the NAMES Project serendipitously planted me directly in front of a quilt panel I had made years before for John. Providing drinking water to the AIDS Ride bicyclists as they crossed the midwestern prairies sent me into dreams in which the heavy sandbags holding down our tents were filled with human ashes. Joining a die-in on the White House lawn brought some closure. Yes, I prayed there too. We fell to the ground when the signal came, after we had encircled the White House three deep, holding hands and singing. We all prayed there.

I've seen buffalo in a North Dakota blizzard, sat quietly near empty sweat lodges adding mental prayer ties to their rounded frames. I've let grief and tension stream out of the pores of my torso in a healing massage and allowed a stranger to hold me on a field in Washington, DC, when the quilt made its first appearance. I've walked many labyrinths, one that I shared with a cow, heard Tibetan chanting in a Unitarian church, gone to Passover seders in several midwestern homes, celebrated the Romanian government's overthrow with immigrant St. Paulites.

I've prayed through the changing seasons of tall Wisconsin hardwoods during a five-hour daily commute to visit my brain-injured mother. I've prayed while tossing imaginary pieces of paper holding names of the dead into predawn bonfires. I've prayed during water rituals with women who were also sexually abused. I prayed as I cleaned out the San Francisco apartment of a neighbor who killed himself. I whispered prayers when I found out that Casey had become an alcoholic and had stopped eating. And I prayed later when she died, myself too ill to attend her memorial. I've found spiritual meaning through my photography by capturing places of memory, beauty, and serenity.

No, I haven't spent a lot of time in churches, although for years I never felt it was really Christmas until after I stood in a circle with the guys down at the AIDS Project reciting the Lord's Prayer during their annual holiday gathering. My most healing church experiences were in a tiny four-person chapel open 24/7 in DC and at a poetry reading by Carolyn Forché in the sanctuary of St. Stephen's Church.

My prayers were also grateful ones. That I found some words to say, that I didn't fall asleep at the wheel, that I was able to carry on with complicated duties of guardianship of my brother, of probate and the selling of a new home my mother had lived in for only six months. Joyful ones for the saving of a handful of men from all those I knew in San Francisco, including Tim, now a flourishing artist who continues to inspire me. Grateful ones for new pen pals from among my dead friends' family members and former lovers. The borrowed time to whisper and touch a sweating brow. That Elizabeth was able to buy a small house, that Kim and Jon's still stands and that they continue to include me in their lives. The miracle of my reunion with Neal, months before he died of leukemia at age fifty-one. That Phil found his true love in New York as Leon had in Oregon. For the countless friendships in the Minnesota AIDS movement—a loving community who took me in and helped me heal (Ford, Brian, Deb, Greg and Rob, Dick, Pat, and countless others, some who are no longer alive). I said grateful prayers for deep experiences in support groups, on committees, with a grief group, with volunteers.

For the sparing of my own life and the continual recovery from survivor's guilt, and mostly for the bright years with my San Francisco pals in those elusive days of our youth. These are the things I refuse to relinquish. No politician, policeman, or homophobic protester can take them. These memories are for me and for those of us who remain.

CPSIA information can be obtained
at www.ICGtesting.com
Printed in the USA
LVHW04s0109130918
590006LV00013B/157/P

9 781732 284500